Topics in Mining, Metallurgy and Materials Engineering

Series editor

Carlos P. Bergmann, Porto Alegre, Brazil

"Topics in Mining, Metallurgy and Materials Engineering" welcomes manuscripts in these three main focus areas: Extractive Metallurgy/Mineral Technology; Manufacturing Processes, and Materials Science and Technology. Manuscripts should present scientific solutions for technological problems. The three focus areas have a vertically lined multidisciplinarity, starting from mineral assets, their extraction and processing, their transformation into materials useful for the society, and their interaction with the environment.

More information about this series at http://www.springer.com/series/11054

Venina dos Santos · Rosmary Nichele Brandalise
Michele Savaris

Engineering of Biomaterials

Springer

Venina dos Santos
UCS
Caxias do Sul, Rio Grande do Sul
Brazil

Michele Savaris
UCS
Caxias do Sul, Rio Grande do Sul
Brazil

Rosmary Nichele Brandalise
UCS
Caxias do Sul, Rio Grande do Sul
Brazil

ISSN 2364-3293 ISSN 2364-3307 (electronic)
Topics in Mining, Metallurgy and Materials Engineering
ISBN 978-3-319-58606-9 ISBN 978-3-319-58607-6 (eBook)
DOI 10.1007/978-3-319-58607-6

Library of Congress Control Number: 2017940235

Printed on acid-free paper

This Springer imprint is published by Springer Nature
The registered company is Springer International Publishing AG
The registered company address is: Gewerbestrasse 11, 6330 Cham, Switzerland

Preface

The use of biomaterials has substantially increased in the last decades. This occurs due to population aging, life expectancy increasing and lifestyle, and implants technology improvements. The development of biomaterials with necessary characteristics to aid in tissue recovery caused by accident or disease is one of the biggest challenges in the scientific field, which involves biomedical and engineering areas. The most important factor that differentiates a biomaterial of other material is the ability to be in contact with human body tissues without causing damages of unacceptable magnitude. The biomaterial must be biocompatible, biofunctional, inert, and sterilizable. They are classified according to their chemical nature, as metal, ceramic, polymeric, and composites. Metallic materials are used because of their good mechanical strength properties, high toughness, easy manufacture, and low cost. Ceramic materials have low electrical and thermal conductivity and exhibit good chemical stability. Polymeric materials are used because of physico-chemical characteristics and structural versatility. Composite materials are used because of specific properties obtained only when different types of materials are combined.

This book contains an updated overview of Engineering of Biomaterials. Its content includes case studies of application of biomaterials and provides in a clear and objective manner a context of biomaterials within areas of knowledge like medicine, physiotherapy, biology, chemistry, materials science, chemical engineering, and mechanical engineering. The authors have practical experience with manufacturing processes of metal, polymer, and ceramic artifacts, degradation of polymeric materials in vitro tests and sterilization processes. This book is addressed to students, researchers, doctors, physiotherapists, and engineers who search for a deeper general knowledge in biomaterials. I am sure that the clear language and the application-oriented perspective of this book will widely satisfy the readers' exigencies.

Porto Alegre, Brazil
March 2017

Carlos P. Bergmann

Contents

Chapter 1
Introduction

As we grow old, our articulations become arthritic, bones turn fragile and break, teeth start to wear out, hearing and vision are reduced or lost, the circulatory system gives signs of being blocked, the heart loses control of its rhythm and pumping, valves lose their sealing capacity, tumors appear in bones, breasts, skin, and vital organs. Besides, the ability to maim, crush, break, and disfigure the human body with vehicles, fire arms, drugs, tools, or through practicing sports is inherent to human beings [1].

On the other hand, as pointed out by scientists, the oldest human being ever is already born, outweighing the 122 years of the French woman Jeanne Calment. Some of the factors which contribute to the rise of population number are the higher longevity of the population and the high birth rate in some countries. It is estimated that more than 893 million people are older than 60 years. Up to the end of the twenty-first century according to the United Nations (UN), this figure will triple, reaching 2.4 billion. The average life span in 2016 was 68 years.

The quest for improvements in quality of life and the rise in life expectation has rendered possible to modern society to witness scientific and technological progress in various fields during the past few years. Relevant medical progress, but above all, progress in engineering has enabled solutions for many current day problems through the development of a new category of materials, the so-called Biomaterials. In accordance with the 1992 Conference on Biomaterials for clinical applications, by biomaterials is meant every material (except drugs) or combination or materials, of synthetic or natural original, which for an undetermined period of time is employed as the whole or an integral portion of a system for treatment, enlargement, or replacement of any tissues, organs, or body functions [2, 3].

At this same Conference, in 1987, by virtue of the development of these materials and interface technologies with the biologic medium, biomaterials are developed aiming at interacting with biologic systems, treat, and increase or replace any tissue, organ, or function of the human body, being artificially produced or modified [3].

V. dos Santos et al., *Engineering of Biomaterials*, Topics in Mining, Metallurgy and Materials Engineering, DOI 10.1007/978-3-319-58607-6_1

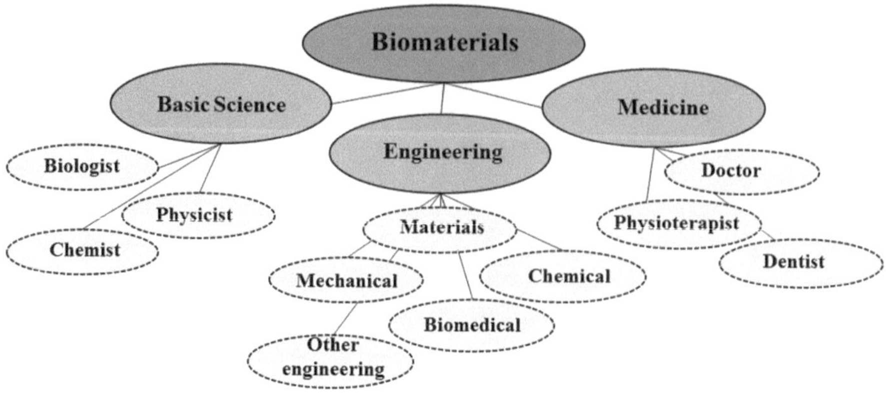

Fig. 1.1 Schematic representation of the interdisciplinary areas of biomaterials

Understanding the complex interactions between Biomaterials, made up of different kinds of materials and their combinations and living tissues becomes a challenge for the fields of basic sciences (Biology, Physics, and Chemistry), engineering, and medicine (Fig. 1.1).

Turning back to history, Biomaterials are mentioned not as recent developments. On this 3000-year-old mummy, there is evidence that an ancient Egyptian physician crafted this prosthesis to help an ailing patient—in this case, a 50–60-year-old woman whose toe had been amputated or lost in an accident. The biomaterial that he used was wood. Historically biomaterials were common knowledge for doctors and priests, gold was used as dental repair by Chinese, Aztecs, and Romans 2000 years ago. In 1775, iron and brass were already used for the restoration of a fractured femur. The first glass eye was produced in 1832 by the Ludwig Müller-Uri glass blower in Lauscha, Germany. Indigenous populations of Central America and Africa made use of ants' clamps for sewing wounds, besides, George Washington (1732–1799) had cow, hypo, and ivory teeth manufactured by his dentist John Greenwood in 1793 hinged by a metal frame with an opening spring. It is said the George Washington does not look comfortable in the US one dollar bill because of the pain caused by his false teeth, it is speculated that the spring mechanism required much effort to keep the mouth closed, this being expressed on his face stamped on the one dollar bill [4].

Failure of the first materials acting as Biomaterials was due to the lack of attention devoted to the biological suitability of same. A contemporary approach is distinguished by the rational development of materials for the production of medical devices based on a better understanding of their function and of the interface between the material and the environment where the device is supposed to work. The "in vivo" environment is not static, life is not a stable condition it is a dynamic metastable process which constantly exchanges energy and material with the outer world in order to produce work. An efficient device should be manufactured from a material which does not bring disorder to the metastable process of the living being or the performance of the device in the environment where it is going to be inserted for an undetermined period of time.

The introduction of implants in the human body can activate the immune system, yielding systemic symptoms such as asthma, hives, and hypersensitivity to a certain material, which can lead to tissue necrosis by local vascular thrombosis.

Biomaterials can be classified in different ways according to the response of the tissue/body to the implant: in case the tissues die, the material is considered toxic, if it forms a fibrous tissue, the material is considered inert, if it promotes an interfacial link, it is considered bioactive and, finally, if it promotes the tissue replacement, the material is considered soluble [5].

In the beginning of the use of biomaterials in a more systematic way, in the fifties, the search was focused on bioinert materials. As time went by, the search was directed to the bioactivity of materials, and more recently, the focus has been on the regeneration of a true functional tissue, the focus being on the response of the body and not on that of the biomaterial, which is to perform the function to which it has been designed with the minimum biological response of the patient.

In the course of time, efforts were devoted to increasing the useful life of the implant through its interaction with the interface of the host tissue, then, the focus was directed to the development of biodegradable materials, able to be incorporated or absorbed (after dissolution) by the host tissue, and more recently, the concept of biomimetics, searching for materials which would participate actively in the recovery process, working on the tissue in a specific way, with stimulation at the cell level [6].

The evolution in the development and utilization of biomaterials is illustrated in Fig. 1.2 [7].

There are several steps involved since the identification of the requirements and needs of a biomaterial, its utilization, and up to the final response of product and host.

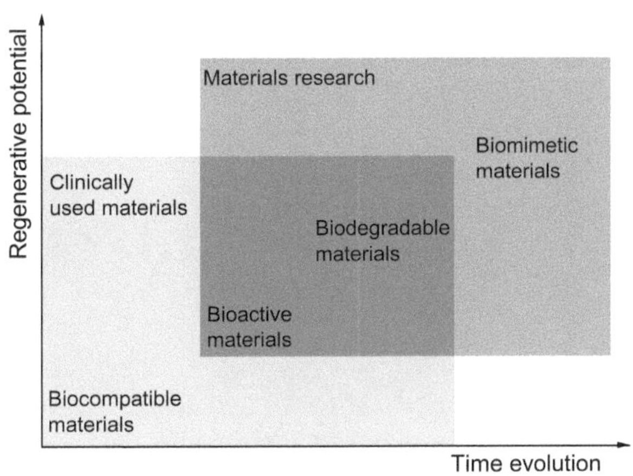

Fig. 1.2 Evolution in the development and utilization of biomaterials. Adapted [7]

Biomaterials are made up of different classifications of materials: metallic, ceramic and polymeric and composites. These classifications, among others, will be approached in the next chapters of this book.

More than any other area of the current technique, the field of biomaterials as a science requires that interdisciplinary teams work together, with researchers of different fields in the search for the development of innovative biomaterials, adaptable or suitable to individuals under growth, as well as new technologies for their production and characterization, with a relevant role in the field and which will require huge efforts and investments [4].

References

1. Hench, L.L.: Biomaterials: a forecast for the future. Biomaterials **19**(16), 1419–1423 (1998)
2. Nicholson, J.W.: The Chemistry of Medical and Dental Materials. Royal Society of Chemistry, Cambridge (2002)
3. Williams, D.F.: On the mechanisms of biocompatibility. Biomaterials **29**, 2941–2953 (2008)
4. Pires, A.L.R., Bierhalz, A.C.K.E., Moraes, Â.M.: Biomateriais: tipos, aplicações e mercado. Quim. Nova **38**(7), 957–971 (2015)
5. Oréfice, R.L.: Biomateriais, fundamentos e aplicações. Cultura Médica, Rio de Janeiro (2006)
6. Ratner, B.D., Hoffman, A.S., Schoen, F.J., Lemons, J.E.: Biomaterials Science: An Introduction to Materials in Medicine, 3rd edn. Academic Press, Amsterdam (2013)
7. Holzapfel, B.M., Reichert, J.C., Schantz, J.T., Gbureck, U., Rackwitz, L., Noth, U., Jakob, F., Rudert, M., Groll, J., Hutmacher, D.W.: How smart do biomaterials need to be? A translational science and clinical point of view. Adv. Drug Deliv. Rev. **65**(4), 581–603 (2013)

Chapter 2
Biomaterials: Characteristics and Properties

The design and selection of a biomaterial depend on its specific application in order to be useful and assure its properties as long as required, without rejection [1]. In order to be considered a biomaterial it should, besides not inducing inflammation, toxic reactions and allergenic symptoms in the body, be biocompatible, biofunctional, bioactive, bioinert and sterilizable (Fig. 2.1) [2, 3].

A further condition for a biomaterial is that the processes of hygienization and sterilization should not promote modifications in the properties of same [3].

The biomaterial surface, being directly exposed to the living organism, plays a crucial role as regards biocompatibility. When this issue is considered, the physical, morphological, and biologic characteristics can be adapted to promote improvement in the interaction of biomaterial and tissue [2].

The concept of biocompatibility has been deeply altered in these last few years. At first it was believed that a material was biocompatible by being completely inert to the human body, without any response from the biological medium to its presence. The idea of a totally inert material was abandoned when it could be observed that the presence of any kind of material always entails some response from the body, varying as a function of the kind of application and the patients' characteristics (age, sex, etc.). Thus, the concept of biocompatibility of a material, by emphasizing especially the tissue (or neighboring medium) material interface, could be defined only by encompassing the various forms of interaction of the body with the material [4].

Biomaterials can be utilized for various applications in a myriad of areas of the human body. However, for each of these applications, the commonly required feature is the degree of tolerance of these biomaterials when in contact with organs and tissues. In order to comply with this aspect, the biomaterials should undergo critical adjustments so as to serve each specific application in the best possible way. One mode of adjusting the surface characteristics of the biomaterials is by means of surface modifications, which keep the characteristics of internal properties of the material with a suitable surface in order to better meet the specification of the locus of application.

V. dos Santos et al., *Engineering of Biomaterials*, Topics in Mining, Metallurgy and Materials Engineering, DOI 10.1007/978-3-319-58607-6_2

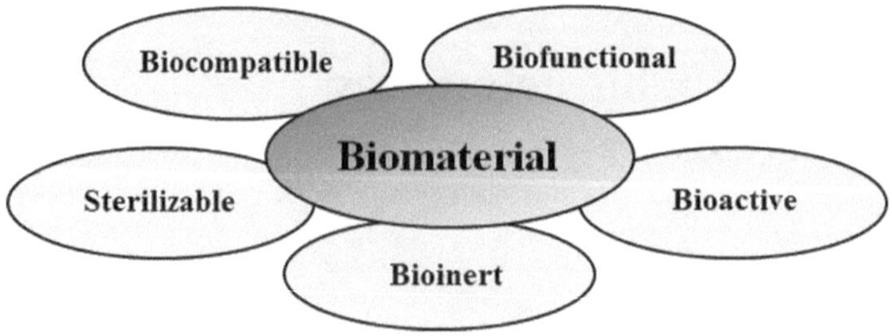

Fig. 2.1 Characteristics that a material must present to be a biomaterial

The use of medical implants increased in the last decades due to the population aging, boost in life expectancy and style of life and improvements in implant technology [5].

The development of biomaterials having the required characteristics to aid in the recovery of tissues damaged by accidents or disease is one of the major challenges in the scientific field involving medical and engineering areas [6].

Every material used as a biomaterial in the medical field, either by organ replacement, support for tissue growth or drug release should have specific characteristics in order not to stimulate or cause any level of allergenic or inflammatory response to the human body. The characteristics to be taken into consideration when it is meant a biomaterial used for implant include biocompatibility, biofunctionality, chemical, and mechanical stability. Besides these characteristics, the material should be sterilizable in order to avoid irritation, rejection, and/or problems at the locus of implant [7, 8].

Biocompatibility of a biomaterial as previously defined is related to the organism accepting the body, until then a foreign matter, and admitting it as part of the whole, as well as not exhibiting signs of harmful effects at its locus of operation. The expression biocompatibility comprehends different properties of materials, such as toxicity, tissues compatibility, blood compatibility (hemocompatibility), and biofunctionality properties [9].

Biofunctionality is essential for the material to perform the functions to which it has been designed for, at the required period of time and effectively. For materials of long-lasting biofunctionality the material should not degrade by contact with the tissue; since thus it would partly lose its functionality, it should also keep its chemical and mechanical stability throughout the whole process to which it has been enabled. For metals, degradation is related to corrosion which causes harmful effects to the body if these are not of a tolerable degree [4, 7].

As for the response of the body, biomaterials can be characterized as biotolerable, bioinert, bioactive, and biodegradable [10].

Biotolerable is the way by which are designed materials that are tolerated by the body, being separated from the host tissue by the formation of a housing of fibrous tissue. This layer is induced by the release of chemical compounds, ions, corrosion products, and other ones resulting from the implanted material. Among the biotolerable materials are highlighted the synthetic polymer materials and most of the metals [10].

Bioinert are materials which are also tolerated by the body, but where there is no chemical reaction between the material and the tissue. The material either does not release components in any significant amount or does not release components and the formation of fibrous housing is minimal. Common examples of bioinert materials are alumina, zirconia, titanium and alloys and carbon [10].

Bioactive are materials that can make chemical bonds with the bone tissue, characterized as an osseointegration process. Through this process the bone tissue connects to the implanted material promoting the coating by bone cells. Materials employed as bioactive are the calcium phosphate, hydroxyapatite, and calcium phosphate compound-based glasses and vitroceramics [10].

Biodegradable are materials which degrade, solubilize, or are absorbed when in contact with the body for a certain period of time. Their application is of deep interest since there is no need of a further surgery for the withdrawal of the implant. Within this class most important are the biopolymers [10].

A biomaterial which otherwise complies with all the characteristics required for its utilization can only be effectively employed if it can be sterilized. Sterilization is crucial since it is by means of this procedure that all impurities and microorganisms are eliminated, providing a material which is suitable for implant [11, 12].

According to regulating authorities such as the Therapeutic Goods Administration (TGA), Food and Drug Administration (FDA), European Commission on Health and Consumers (ECHC), and Medical Devices Bureau of Health Canada, medical devices are classed following their complexity and required control level to assure safety and effectiveness. In Australia, besides the cited classification is also attributed a class according to the degree of invasiveness and onto which tissue the device is applied to (e.g., class III corresponds to chronic diseases implantable devices). Non-implant (class I and II) medical devices (e.g., surgical and dental instruments) are manufactured from commercial-grade materials (Table 2.1). Biomaterials of higher interest for the scientific community can be found in the higher classes of Table 2.1, with characteristics suitable for prolonged contact with human tissues and thus require premarket approval [1].

The choice of the biomaterial is associated with the function it will perform and the period of time it will contact the human body, based on the combination of its physical, chemical, mechanical, and biological properties [13, 14].

2.1 Properties of Biomaterials

The biomaterial success for a certain application is related, besides the specific items for biomaterials cited above, to its physical, chemical, and mechanical properties. According to the effort demanded from the material and the region to which it will be applied, such properties can be modified and thus they deserve careful attention when choosing a material.

Table 2.1 Some accepted classifications and description of medical devices [1]

Authority	Class			
TGA	I	IIa, IIb	III	–
FDA	I	II	III	–
ECHC	I	IIa	IIb	III
Health Canada	I	II	III	IV
Description				
General description	Non invasive and/or transient use (e.g., dermal)	Minimally invasive, short term (e.g., eyes, ear canal)	Short to medium term contact with blood, oral/nasal mucosae	Medium to long term contact, chronic implants, control systems
Restrictions	General	General and specific	General control and premarket approvals	–
Health risk	Low	Low/moderate	Moderate/high	High
Example	Surgical instruments, mechanical barriers	Contact lenses, ultrasound probes	Orthopedic implants, dialysis machines	Pacemakers, perfusion pumps, vascular stents

2.1.1 Physical Properties

The physical properties of the biomaterial are fundamental for the response of cell adhesion. When cells adhere to the biomaterial surface physical chemical reactions between cell and biomaterial occur, such reactions being influenced by factors such as cell behavior, biomaterial surface properties, and environmental factors. The biomaterial surface properties include wettability, filler, roughness, softness, and chemical composition [15].

Wettability (hydrophobicity/hydrophilicity) is one of the parameters affecting the biological response of the biomaterial and describes the balance between the solid surface intermolecular interactions with a liquid. Among the affected properties are protein adsorption, platelet adhesion/activation, blood coagulation, and cellular and bacterial adhesion. Hydrophobic surfaces are, generally, considered as more protein-adsorbent than hydrophilic surfaces due to the hydrophobic interactions occurring at the surface in contrast with the solvation forces which are water repellent relative to the water linked to the hydrophilic surface [16].

As relates to surface charge, researchers reported improved biocompatibility, cellular affinity, and cellular differentiation on surfaces of biomaterials implanted utilizing positive ions and negative ions. For example, 2-hydroxyethyl methacrylate (HEMA) gels incorporated with positive charges promoted better adhesion and spreading of fibroblasts and osteoblasts when compared with negative or neutral charges [15].

The roughness of the biomaterial also plays an important role in the adhesion and cellular behavior and exerts direct influence both in vitro and in vivo. Smooth surface and rough surface have different contact areas with molecules and cells and this difference in contact influences the kind of biological units' links and therefore, conformation and function. In most of the cases cells prefer rough surface to smooth ones, due to the fact that rough surfaces favor proliferation [15].

For low friction applications, such as in implants of orthopedic joints, biomaterials with mirrored finishes are preferred. And when tissue-implant integration is desired, as is the case of endobone implants, high roughness is preferred [17].

The surface roughness of a biomaterial should be studied in terms of amplitude and organization. Studies revealed that low-amplitude surface grooves induce orientation of groups of cells or individual cells along its axis this being the basis to state that the best parameter for the orientation of cells would be the groove's width and not its depth. Still, oriented osteoblasts tend to mineralize more quickly, favoring the tissue/implant osseointegration process [18]. Still, for cases where the biomaterial is used for dental implants, high roughness surfaces could show risks of increased peri-implantitis, peri-implantar mucositis, or ionic release in case of alloys [19].

Case Study: Relationship between surface properties (roughness, wettability) of titanium and titanium alloys and cell behavior [20]

A study performed on a titanium-based biomaterial reports data on wettability, surface free energy, interfacial free energy, and roughness aiming at determining which of these parameters had the strongest influence on the response of human fibroblasts proliferation.

Titanium samples contained neat titanium (Cp-Ti), titanium–aluminum–vanadium alloy (Ti–6Al–4V) and titanium–nickel (Ni–Ti). Ni–Ti had different roughness values, Ni–Ti80 (Ra = 1.02 ± 0.17 μm), Ni–Ti400 (Ra = 0.15 ± 0.015 μm), and Ni–Ti2400 (Ra = 0.057 ± 0009 μm), Ti–6Al–4V (Ra = 0.068 ± 0.007 μm), and Cp-Ti (Ra = 0.064 ± 0.008 μm). Upon evaluation of cellular proliferation at the several roughness values, results indicated that cells showed preference for surface roughness values lower than 1 μm.

Wettability was evaluated for the rough surfaces and for smooth surfaces. For rough surfaces wettability exhibited higher contact angle for the highest roughness sample (Ni–Ti80), both in the parallel (69 ± 11°) and in the perpendicular (73 ± 5°) direction. For smooth surfaces of the Cp-Ti, Ni–Ti, and Ti–6Al–4V samples with roughness below 0.015 μm (mechanical polish), the contact angle with water was of hydrophilic nature with close values for Cp-Ti (53.9 ± 5.1°) and Ti–6Al–4V (50 ± 3.1°) and higher values for Ni–Ti (60.4 ± 5.8°), proliferation being bigger at the Ni–Ti surface.

In accordance with the Owens–Wendt calculations, the total surface free energy was 46 ± 3 mJ/m^2 for Ni–Ti and 52 ± 2 mJ/m^2 for Cp-Ti and Ti–6Al–4V. As regards fibroblasts proliferation, it was bigger for the Ni–Ti sample, this being possibly related to the lower value of total surface free energy. Interfacial free energy had extremely low values (Ni–Ti: 2.36 ± 0.15 mJ/m^2, Cp-Ti: 2.4 ± 0.05 mJ/m^2, Ti–6Al–4V: 2.17 ± 0.07 mJ/m^2) which could be attributed to hydrogel formation at the metal surface.

The study evidenced that roughness influences human fibroblasts proliferation, as well as the wettability characteristic. However, surface free energy can be a dominant parameter for fibroblasts proliferation.

2.1.2 Chemical Properties

The physical properties, composition, and chemical properties also influence the kind of cell bond and determine the biomaterial chemical stability and reactivity.

The corporeal ambience is harsh and may cause corrosion of biomaterials. On account of this fact, the biomaterials' chemical stability becomes a relevant factor as regards biocompatibility.

Corrosion products may cause adverse reactions to the implant neighborhood. Body fluids are in balance with specific ions under normal physiological conditions. When a biomaterial is implanted the concentration of these ions increases significantly around it and may cause swelling and pain, besides the fact that the corrosion wastes may migrate to other parts of the body and cause undesirable reactions, both for the tissues and the implant [21].

Corrosion of biomaterials alters not only chemical stability, but also affects the mechanical integrity, with possible premature failure of the material [21].

As with corrosion, the corporeal ambience may cause and/or accelerate the biomaterial degradation. Degradation can also be influenced by sterilization processes to which materials are submitted [22–24]. When the biomaterial is degraded, modifications occur at the material structure and, consequently, modifications in its properties.

Surface functional groups can also influence the biomaterial response, since the surface chemical functionality affects adsorbed protein and cell/protein interactions. Commonly investigated functionalities as relates biomaterials are carboxyl (–COOH), hydroxyl (–OH), amino (–NH_2), and methyl (–CH_3) groups [25].

2.1.3 Mechanical Properties

Advances in engineering and medicine require the development of ever more specialized properties for biomaterials. For a biomaterial utilized for a specific mechanical application, some of the requirements studied are Young's modulus, ductility, tensile strength, yield strength, compression strength and fatigue, and wear debris. These properties are evaluated on account of the fact that the human body has different properties for each tissue. For example, elasticity varies from very soft as is the case of brain tissues ($\sim$0.1–1 kPa) up to extremely hard or stiff (30 kPa and above), which is the case for the completely mineralized bone [26].

Biomaterials having Young's modulus close to that of the bone are recommended since they assure uniform tensile distribution and avoid stress shielding after implant placement; high values for yield and compression strength properties avoid fractures and improve functional stability; ductility is important for modeling the biomaterial formation and for dental biomaterials. The ductility minimum value is 8%; hardness and tenacity also evaluate the biomaterial response; the increase in hardness reduces the wear incidence; and increase in tenacity renders fracture more difficult [27]. These features, besides defining the processing ability of the biomaterial, are used to evaluate the success and biocompatibility of same.

Still as relates mechanical properties, biomaterials used for hip implant or articulation replacement should bear cyclic loads without failure or fracture for a long period of time, the same being true for cardiac valves. Besides numerous cyclic loads, failure by fatigue can also occur if tensile variations are high [2]. Biomaterials which should bear cyclic efforts without allowing cracking propagation are made up chiefly of polyurethane, polyester, and metals in general. The biomaterials which bear the desired characteristics are mainly applied for orthopedic, dental, and cardiovascular implants [17].

Wear causes material surface removal and this process occurs by the movement of two surfaces in contact. Failure by fatigue and wear can occur, for example, in biomaterials used for hip prosthesis, where the contact movement of the biomaterial parts is imperative. Besides, the physiological medium may aggravate these phenomena [2].

Biomaterials used for replacement of intervertebral disk should have fair properties of compression strength since the backbone undergoes compression caused by the body weight besides those due to the contraction loads of the muscles surrounding the backbone. For example, compression forces during dynamic lifting were estimated in up to 2500 N and the intradiscal pressure of approximately 1 MPa during routine activities, such as climbing steps (0.5–0.7 MPa) and jogging (0.35–0.95 MPa) [28]. Table 2.2 lists the load applied in different activities on the lumbar intervertebral disk (L-3) for a 70 kg individual [29].

Differentiated cells or stem cells of different organs and tissues of the body can feel the properties of biomaterials, such as the matrix elasticity and convey the mechanical signs as physiological responses, such as strain specification, cell orientation, morphological alterations, and growth factor. The development of bio-adaptive materials having mechanical properties similar to those of damaged tissues or organs could favor cell adaptation [30].

Table 2.2 Load applied on the intervertebral disk as related to different activities [29]

Activity	Load on disk (N)
Supine position	294
Standing	686
Seated right	980
Walking	833
Rolling the trunk	882
Inclining laterally	931
Coughing	1078
Jumping	1078
Stretching out	1176
Laughing	1176
Lifting 20 kg with upright column, flexed knees	2058
Lifting 20 kg with bent column, stretched knees	3332

2.2 Surface Modification—Biomaterial–Tissue Interactions

Modifications at the biomaterial surfaces are considered as a promising alternative to improve biomaterial–tissue interactions and promote better biocompatibility and biofunctionality results without altering the materials' bulk properties [31].

Surface modifications can be of the following kinds: physicochemical modifications (related to modifications involving changes of atoms, constituents, or surface molecules) and surface coating (involving different materials for underlying support). Physical–chemical modifications can be obtained by means of chemical reactions (oxidation, reduction, utilization of organosilanes, acetylation), etching, mechanical roughening/polishing, and patterning; and surface coatings include grafting, non-covalent, and covalent coating, besides thin film deposition [31]. Figure 2.2 illustrates a few surface modification techniques.

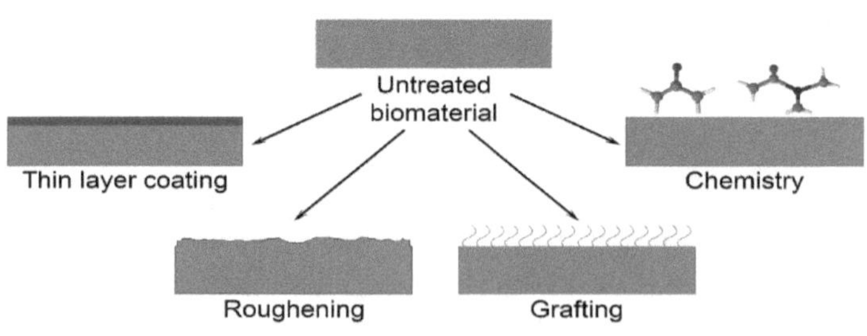

Fig. 2.2 Illustration of surface modification techniques for biomaterials

Table 2.3 Different techniques and coating characteristics with apatite deposition

Technique	Thickness	Advantages	Disadvantages
Thermal spraying	30–200 μm	High deposition rates, low cost	Line of sight technique, high temperatures induce decomposition, rapid cooling
Sputter coating	0.5–3 μm	Uniform coating thickness on flat substrates, dense coating	Line of sight technique, expensive time consuming, produces amorphous coatings
Dip coating	0.05–0.5 mm	Inexpensive, coatings applied quickly, can coat complex substrates	High sintering temperature, thermal expansion mismatch
Sol–gel	<1 μm	Can coat complex shapes, low processing temperature, relatively cheap as coatings are very thin	Process require controlled atmosphere processing, expensive raw materials
Electrophoretic deposition	0.1–2.0 mm	Uniform coating thickness, rapid deposition rates, can coat complex substrates	Difficult to produce crack-free coatings, requires high sintering temperatures
Pulsed laser deposition	0.05–5 μm	Coating with crystalline and amorphous, coating with dense and porous	Line of sight technique
Biomimetic coating	<30 μm	Low processing temperatures, can form bonelike apatite, can coat complex shapes, can incorporate bone growth stimulating factors	Requires replenishment and a constant pH of simulated body fluid

Adapted [32]

In the group of coatings those listed in Table 2.3 are highlighted. These surface coatings are obtained by deposition of hydroxyapatite, a bioactive material which favors the osseointegration process [32, 33].

A huge variety of techniques for surface modifications is to be found in the literature; however, no universal technique is known that could be used for any type of biomaterial. What are known are process variations and those depend on the desired application and the kind of biomaterial. For example, for bone implant biomaterial quick bone conductivity is required and stents should be structured to avoid cell proliferation provoking restenosis, while a cardiovascular device should have blood compatibility or antithrombogenicity [34].

The choice of the surface modification technique is a function of factors such as the substrate material, components and geometry design, application and surface aspects of engineering processes which include coating thickness and process temperature [34].

References

1. Chen, Q., Thouas, G.A.: Metallic implant biomaterials. Mat. Sci. Eng. R. **87**, 1–57 (2015)
2. Bauer, S., Schmuki, P., Von Der Mark, K., Park, J.: Engineering biocompatible implant surfaces Part I: materials and surfaces. Prog. Mater Sci. **58**, 261–326 (2013)
3. Domanska, A., Boczkowska, A.: Biodegradable polyurethanes from crystalline prepolymers. Polym. Degrad. Stab. **108**, 175–181 (2014)
4. Oréfice, R.L., Pereira, M. de. M., Mansur, H.S.: Biomateriais: fundamentos e eaplicações. Cultura Médica, Rio de Janeiro (2006)
5. Holzapfel, B.M., Reichert, J.C., Schantz, J.T., Gbureck, U., Rackwitz, L., Noth, U., Jakob, F., Rudert, M., Groll, J., Hutmacher, D.W.: How smart do biomaterials need to be? A translational science and clinical point of view. Adv. Drug Deliv. Rev. **65**, 581–603 (2013)
6. Lasprilla, A.J.R., Martinez, G.A.R., Lunelli, B.H., Jardini, A.L., Maciel Filho, R.: Poly-lactic acid synthesis for application in biomedical devices: a review. Biotechnol. Adv. **30**(1), 321–328 (2012)
7. Ravaglioli, A., Krajewski, A.: Bioceramics—Materials, Proprieties Applications. Chapman & Hall, Nova York (1992)
8. Silver, F., Doillon, C.: Biocompatibility: interactions of biological and implantable materials. VCH, New York (1989)
9. Wang, Y.X., Robertson, J.L., Spillman Jr., W.B., Claus, R.O.: Effects of the chemical structure and the surface properties of polymeric biomaterials on their biocompatibility. Pharm. Res. **21**(8), 1362–1373 (2004)
10. Hench, L.L., Wilson, J.: An Introduction to Bioceramics. World Scientific Publish, Singapore (1999)
11. Rai, R., Tallawi, M., Roether, J.A., Detsch, R., Barbani, N., Rosellini, E., Kaschta, J., Schubert, D.W., Boccaccini, A.R.: Sterilization effects on the physical properties and cytotoxicity of poly(glycerol sebacate). Mater. Lett. **105**, 32–35 (2013)
12. Ratner, B.D., Hoffman, A.S., Schoen, F.J., Lemons, J.E.: Biomaterials science: an introduction to materials in medicine, 3rd edn. Academic Press, Amsterdam (2013)
13. Kawachi, E.Y., Bertran, C.A., Reis, R.R. dos., Alves, O. L.: Biocerâmics - tendências e perspectivas de uma área interdisciplinar. Quim. Nova. **23**(4), 518–522 (2000)
14. Zuleta, F.A., Velasquez, P., Aza, P.N. de.: Effect of various sterilization methods on the bioactivity of laser ablation pseudowollastonite coating. J. Biomed. Mater. Res. B Appl. Biomater. **94B**(2), 399–405 (2010)
15. Chang, H.I., Wang, Y.: Cell Responses to surface and architecture of tissue engineering scaffolds. In: EBERLI, D. Regenerative Medicine and Tissue Engineering—Cells and Biomaterials, pp. 569–588. INTECH, Croatia (2011)
16. Xu, L.C., Siedlecki, C.A.: Effects of surface wettability and contact time on protein adhesion to biomaterial surfaces. Biomaterials **28**(22), 3273–3283 (2007)
17. da Silva, M.H.P.: Apostila de biomateriais. CBPF, Rio de Janeiro (2006)
18. Wieland, M., Chehroudi, B., Textor, M., Brunette, D.M.: Use of Ti-coated replicas to investigate the effects on fibroblast shape of surfaces with varying roughness and constant chemical composition. J. Biomed. Mater. Res. **60**(3), 434–444 (2002)
19. Chen, W.C., CL, K.O.: Roughened Titanium Surfaces with Silane and Further RGD Peptide Modification in Vitro. Mat. Sci. Eng. C. **33**(5), 2713–22 (2013)
20. Ponsonnet, L., Reybier, K., Jaffrezic, N., Comte, V., Lagneau, C., Lissac, M., Martelet, C.: Relationship between surface properties (roughness, wettability) of titanium and titanium alloys and cell behavior. Mat. Sci. Eng. C. **23**, 551–560 (2003)
21. Smith, W.F., Hashemi, J.: Fundamentos de engenharia e ciência dos materiais, 5th edn. AMGH, Porto Alegre (2012)
22. Holy, C.E., Cheng, C., Davies, J.E., Schoichet, M.: Optimizing the sterilization of PLGA scaffolds for use in tissue engineering. Biomaterials **22**(1), 25–31 (2000)

23. Hooper, K.A., Cox, J.D., Kohn, J. Comparison of the effect of ethylene oxide and g-irradiation on selected tyrosine-derived polycarbonates and poly(L-lactic acid). J. Appl. Polym. Sci. **63**(11), 1499–510 (1997)
24. Loo, S.C.J., Ooi, C.P., Boey, Y.C.F.: Radiation effects on poly(lactide-co-glycolide)(PLGA) and poly(L-lactide) (PLLA). Polym. Degrad. Stab. **83**(2), 259–265 (2004)
25. Thevenot, P., Hu, W., Tang, L.: Surface chemistry influence implant biocompatibility. Curr. Top. Med. Chem. **8**(4), 270–280 (2008)
26. Rehfeldt, F., Engler, A.J., Eckhardt, A., Ahmed, F., Discher, D.E.: Cell responses to the mechanochemical microenvironment: Implications for regenerative medicine and drug delivery. Adv. Drug Deliv. Rev. **59**, 1329–1339 (2007)
27. Saini, M., Singh, Y., Arora, P., Arora, V., Jain, K.: Implant biomaterials: a comprehensive review. World J. Clin. Cases **16**(3), 52–57 (2015)
28. Walter, B.A., Illien-Junger, S., Nasser, P.R., Hencht, A.C., Iatridis, J.C.: Development and validation of a bioreactor system for dynamic loading and mechanical characterization of whole human intervertebral discs in organ culture. J. Biomech. **47**, 2095–2101 (2014)
29. Hamill, J., Kwutzen, K.: Bases biomecânicas do movimento humano. Manole, São Paulo (1999)
30. Wang, Y.: Bioadaptability: an innovative concept for biomaterials. J. Mater. Sci. Technol. **32** (9), 801–809 (2016)
31. Garcia, A.J.: Surface modifications of biomaterials. In: Atala, A., Lanza, R., Thomson, J.A., Nerem, R.M. (eds.) Foundation of Regenerative Medicine, pp. 368–377. Academic Press, San Diego (2010)
32. Yang, Y., Kim, K.H., Ong, J.L.: A review on calcium phosphate coatings produced using a sputtering process—an alternative to plasma spraying. Biomaterials **26**, 327–337 (2005)
33. Ciobanu, G., Ilisei, S., Luca, C.: Hydroxyapatite-silver nanoparticles coatings on porous polyurethane scaffold. Mat. Sci. Eng. C. **35**, 36–42 (2014)
34. Nouri, A., Wen, C.: Introduction to surface coating and modification for metallic biomaterials. In: Wen, C. (ed.) Surface Coating and Modification of Metallic Biomaterials, pp. 3–60. Elsevier Woodhead Publishing, Cambridge (2015)

Chapter 3
Metallic Biomaterials

Biomaterials may be made up of materials of different classifications, such as metallic, ceramic, polymeric and composites.

Among the different raw materials available for the production of biomaterials, metals are highlighted for their good mechanical strength, high tenacity, ease of production and low cost [1, 2].

Metals and their alloys (mixtures or solutions of different metals) have metallic bonds. In this kind of bond the metal atoms organize into a tridimensional ordered arrangement (crystalline structure) in which the valence electrons migrate among atomic centers and form an electronic cloud. Usual crystalline structures present in metals are (a) face-centered cubic (FCC), (b) body-centered cubic (BCC) and (c) hexagonal close packed (HCP) [3–5].

3.1 Development of Metallic Biomaterials

In spite of the huge amount of metals and metallic alloys to be fabricated by industry, only a few are biocompatible and suitable, in the long run, to be employed as biomaterials [5]. The methods of preparation and processing of metals and metallic devices are listed below in Fig. 3.1.

Metals utilized in the biomedical field should be classed into four categories on the basis of the main element of the alloy (Table 3.1): (a) stainless steels, (b) cobalt-based alloys, (c) titanium- and other metals-based alloys (such as for example NiTi and Mg and Ta alloys) [6].

A variety of implants made from metallic materials of the three first groups was approved by the Food and Drug Administration (FDA) [12] of the United States and are usually employed for orthopedic devices [13]. The materials of the last group were recently developed due to their unique properties (such as the NiTi shape memory and the degradability of Mg alloys) which could potentially comply with requirements of more specific tissues [14]. However, some biomaterials

V. dos Santos et al., *Engineering of Biomaterials*, Topics in Mining, Metallurgy and Materials Engineering, DOI 10.1007/978-3-319-58607-6_3

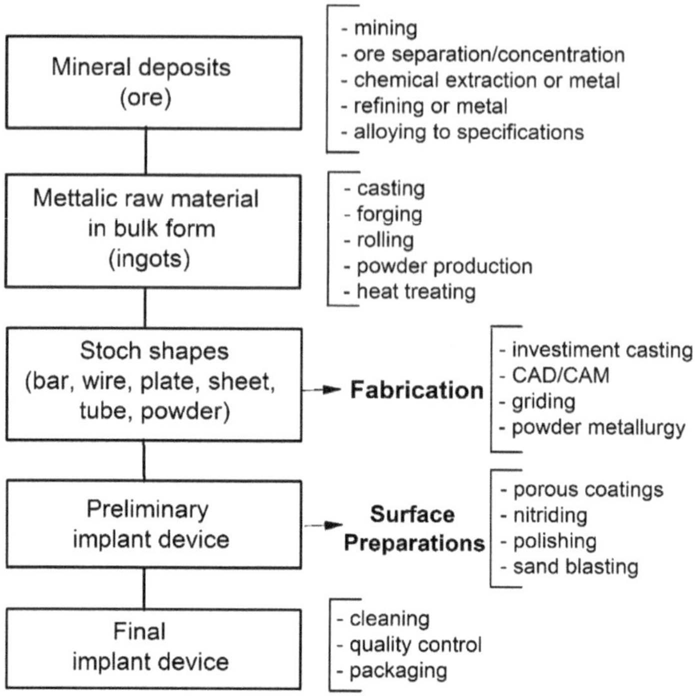

Fig. 3.1 Generic processing of a typical metallic implant device (hip device). Adapted [5]

prepared from these recently developed alloys were not approved by the FDA on account of the problems associated with biocompatibility, which is the main requirement for the application of any biomedical implant [14].

In clinical practice, metal implants are subjected to the conditions as described in Table 3.2 [15].

3.2 Characteristics of Metallic Biomaterials

In order to serve securely and appropriately for a long period of time without rejection, a metallic biomaterial should have the following characteristics [16]:

- Excellent biocompatibility (non-toxic),
- Suitable mechanical properties,
- High corrosion resistance,
- High resistance to wear
- Bone integration (in the case of bone prostheses).

Table 3.1 Four categories of metallic biomaterials and their primary applications as implants [14]

Type	Primary utilizations	Status of applications	References
Stainless steels	1. Temporary devices (fracture plates, screws, hip nails, etc.) (Class II) 2. Total hip replacements (Class II)	Routinely applied	[7]
Co-based alloys	3. Total joint replacement (wrought alloys) (Class II) 4. Dentistry castings (Class II)	Routinely applied	[7]
Ti-based alloys	5. Stem and cup of total hip replacements with CoCrMo or ceramic femoral heads (Class II) 6. Other permanent devices (nails, pacemakers) (Class III)	Routinely applied	[7]
	Miscellaneous others		
NiTi	1. Orthodontic dental archwires (Class I) 2. Vascular stents (Class III) 3. Vena cava filter (Class II) 4. Intracranial aneurysm clips (Class II) 5. Contractile artificial muscles for an artificial heart (Class III) 6. Catheter guide wires (Class II) 7 Orthopedic staples (Class I)	FDA approved FDA approved FDA approved FDA approved Research FDA approved FDA approved	[8]
Mg	8. Biodegradable orthopedic implants (Class III)	Animal trial	[9, 10]
Ta	9. Wire sutures for plastic surgery and neurosurgery (Class III) 10. A radiographic marker (Class II)	FDA approved FDA approved	[11]

3.2.1 Biocompatibility

When developing a biomedical alloy, non-toxic metals should be selected as alloy elements. However, no metal is completely inert or non-toxic. The preparation of metallic biomaterials requires the use of alloys with elements which exist as oligoelements in the body or in the case of reactive alloys, the use of highly corrosion resistant metals (for example, Ti) [16].

3.2.2 Mechanical Properties

Metals properties are regulated by their crystalline structure and by bond strength. High density results from the grouping of atoms into a tridimensional crystalline

Table 3.2 Body environments to which metal implants are subjected [15]

Condition	Parameters	Consequences
Body temperature	37°C	Chemical reaction works faster than in ambient temperature
pH:		
– Blood – Intercelular matrix – Cells	7.15–7.35 7.0 6.8	Even though body fluids are buffered solutions, pH temporary can decrease to ~5.2 around implantation
Dissolved oxygen:		
– Arterial blood – Venous blood – Intercellular matrix	100 mmHg 40 mmHg 2 ~ 40 mmHg	Corrosive environment
Chloride ion:		
– Serum – Interstitial fluid	113 mM 117 mM	Corrosive environment
Mechanical load:		
– Cancellous bone – Cortical bone – Arterial wall – Myocardium – Muscle (max) – Tendon (max	0–4 MPa 0 ~ 40 MPa 0.2–1 MPa 0–0.02 MPa 40 MPa 400 MPa	Could lead to fracture, stress corrosion cracking
Load repetition:		
– Myocardial contraction – Finger joint exercise – Ambulation	$5 \times 10^6 - 4 \times 10^7$/year $10^5 - 10^6$/year 2×10^6/year	Could lead to fatigue, wear and fretting

arrangement, in an ordered and repeated form. The nuclei of positively charged ions are immersed in an electron cloud where they can freely move, being responsible for the good thermal and electrical metals conductivity. Tensile strength results from the intensity of the metallic bonds and the plastic strain occurs due to non-directional bonds, which enable the position of metallic ions to be altered without destroying the crystalline structure [3, 4].

The relevant mechanical properties for the development of biomaterials include Young's modulus, ultimate tensile strength (UTS) and toughness. Such properties of a few metallic biomaterials are presented in Table 3.3 [17]. Stainless steel biomaterials, Co alloys and Ti alloys are widely used on account of their ability to withstand significant loads and undergo plastic strain before failure, such as indicated by their respective UTS and fracture toughness.

One limitation of the metallic biomaterials is related to the value of the metals Young's modulus when compared to that of bones. The ideal situation would be to have an implant the Young modulus of which would be similar to that of bones. According to the values of Table 3.2, the cortical bone Young's modulus varies between 10 and 30 GPa, while for stainless steel and cobalt alloys this value can reach up to 10 times higher [17]. Figure 3.2 illustrates the three orthopedic metallic

Table 3.3 Mechanical Properties of metallic biomaterials and cortical bone [17]

Materials	Young's modulus (GPa)	Ultimate tensile strength (MPa)	Fracture toughness (MPa $\sqrt{m}$)
CoCrMo alloys	240	900–1540	~100
316L stainless steel	200	540–1000	~100
Ti alloys	105–125	900	~80
Mg alloys	40–45	100–250	15–40
NiTi alloys	30–50	1355	30–60
Cortical bone	10–30	130–150	2–12

implants materials (stainless steel, cobalt alloys and titanium and its alloys). In Fig. 3.2 it is possible to observe that these three materials are much stronger and tougher than bone in terms of general mechanical properties and fatigue strength [18]. In cases where the implant Young's modulus is higher than that of bone, the stress shielding phenomenon is likely to occur, as described in Chap. 2, with reduction in bone density and implant loosening causing a chirurgical proceeding for revision. Metals modifications such as pore insertion contribute to make closer the mechanical properties values.

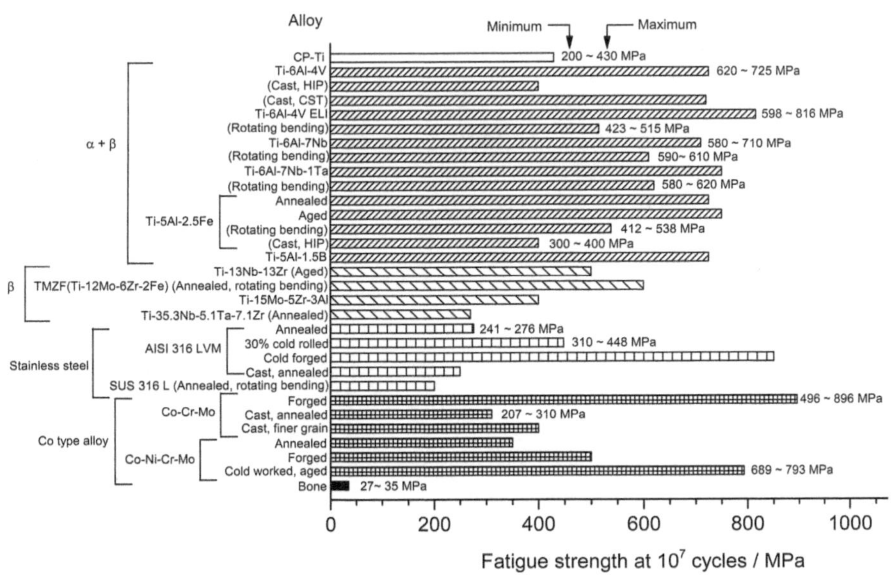

Fig. 3.2 Fatigue strength at 10^7 cycles for biomedical stainless steel, cobalt alloys, titanium and its alloys and bone. Data without designation of rotating bending are those obtained from uniaxial fatigue tests in air [18]

Table 3.4 Typical fatigue mechanical working conditions of some implants [19]

Implants	Loading strength	Loading frequency (Hz)	Expected total number of loading over the life time of a 65 year old patient (i.e. 20 years)
Joints	Compression ~50 MPa	1	10^7
	Bending ~200 MPa	1	10^7
Pacemaker	Not available	1	10^9
Tooth fillings	Not available	1	10^7

Human beings normally walk thousands of paces a day. Under this condition the skeletal bone implants, such as hip prostheses, knee articulations, backbone fixations, plates and wires undergo fatigue caused by cyclic loading (Table 3.4) [19]. This kind of cyclic stress also occurs in dental implants during mastication movement and implants of non-bone tissue such as pacemaker electrodes in response to myocardial activity.

Fatigue strength is related to the maximum intensity of cyclic tension which can be applied to a material without causing failure by fatigue. Fatigue strength varies notably with the materials' microstructure, the product surface quality and the conditions the materials are submitted to, such as, load vectors, cyclic frequency and wear and corrosion environment. A material subject to cyclic loading could fracture well below its UTS and even below the elasticity limit of the material. Fatigue fractures are dangerous since they occur under normal service conditions without prior notice to failure. In order to be able to expect that a medical device manufactured from any material survive to millions of cyclic loadings throughout its useful life it is imperative to perform a thorough exam of fatigue and fracture strength, fracture by fatigue being the main cause of premature failure of biomedical implants. Generally, fatigue starts at a location which acts as a stress concentration area [16].

3.2.3 Corrosion Resistance

Implanted metallic biomaterials keep in contact with body fluids [15]. These media can be aggressive to metals, causing their corrosion. Besides these factors, implants are submitted to the action of mechanical loads which generate friction and sliding, leading to the possible release of metallic particles [4, 20, 21].

Generally speaking, resistance to this corrosion process results from a fine oxide film formed by exposing the metallic surface to air. This film, as a passivation layer, prevents ion exchange, protecting the surface. Some factors, however, can compromise corrosion resistance, such as the lack of homogeneity of the microstructure related to variation in composition, surface deformation, impurities, precipitates, segregations and inclusions. Thus, during the manufacturing process, aiming at improving the corrosion resistance by the strengthening of the protecting film, implants may be submitted to treatments and further oxides deposition on their surface. The favorable side of the metallic implants corrosion resides in using such phenomenon for the development of biodegradable materials of very attractive applications in orthopedic, pediatric and cardiovascular surgeries, where device withdrawal would be rather difficult without damaging the healthy tissue. One of the main metals having potential for this application is magnesium, which has good mechanical properties and low corrosion resistance, its degradation products being quickly excreted from the body and do not exhibit noticeable toxicity. When the availability of materials having controllable corrosion rates is good, it is possible to have implants which dispense with further withdrawal, such as for example vascular stents, screws and rods used in fracture treatments [16].

3.2.4 Wear Resistance

The choice of the kinds of materials for joints depends on the kind of joint. Possible noises can result from friction in metallic implants caused by wear. The occurrence of this problem in patients with hip implants, for example, may reach 10% and usually takes place between 6 month and 2 years after surgery. Wastes cause severe adverse reactions, and a revision surgery is required [22].

High fatigue resistance and excellent wear and corrosion resistance are the main properties which determine the longevity of articulation implants in human body [16].

3.2.5 Osseointegration

Osseointegration is an essential requirement in orthopedics [23]. If the implant surface is not suitably bonded to the bone and other tissues fibrous tissue will form around the implant, causing loosening of the prosthesis [23]. Therefore, it is fundamental for an implant that its surface is suitable for good integration to the neighboring bone. Surface chemistry, surface roughness and surface topography are all factors which should be considered for good osseointegration [24–26].

The selection of the metal used as biomaterial depends on the application. Figure 3.3 illustrates some of the typical locations of clinical use of metallic biomaterials.

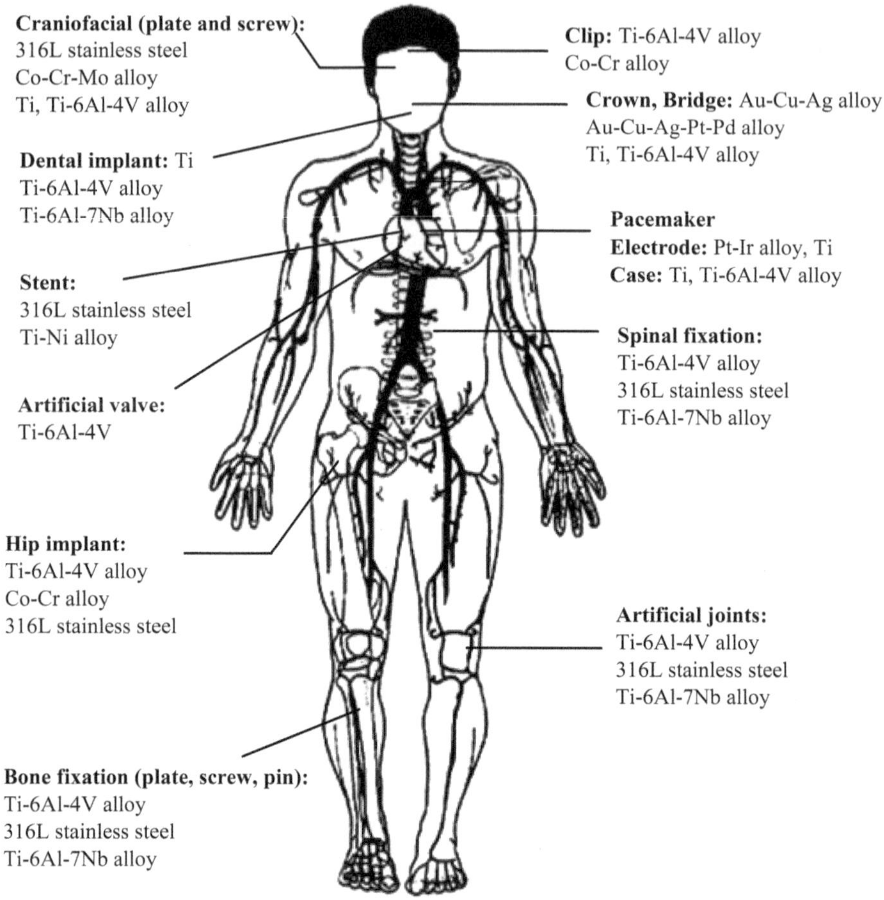

Fig. 3.3 Metallic devices and useful metallic biomaterials. Adapted [27]

3.3 Metallic Biomaterials

The characteristics of some metals usually employed as components of metallic biomaterials are presented below.

3.3.1 Stainless Steel

stainless steels have good mechanical properties, low cost relative to other metals, easy processing e high availability. It is one of the main materials used in fixation devices. These are alloys based on iron, chrome (minimum 12%) and other elements [9, 10].

Steel alloys also have carbon in the structure which can form chrome carbide precipitates on the grain contours, weakening the passivation layer and resulting in lower resistance to corrosion [28]. For biomedical devices low levels of this element are desired, as in austenitic steel 316L, which has a maximum of 0.03% of carbon. This kind of steel is made up of chrome (16–18%), nickel (12–15%) and molybdenum (2–3%). Nickel is added aiming at stabilizing the austenitic structure of iron and improve corrosion resistance. The addition of molybdenum in concentrations above 2% renders the passivation layer more resistant to corrosive media [28].

The use of 316L steel has been challenged on account of the nickel amount, causing toxicity, which can cause problems such as allergies, cancer and genotoxic or mutagenic activities. As a consequence of the adverse effects of nickel release research has been done aiming at developing new stainless steel alloys without this element. The replacement is commonly made by nitrogen, which is a strong stabilizing agent of the austenitic form. The 316L alloy contains from 0.10 to 0.16% nitrogen and has superior wear and corrosion resistance and ductility [29].

3.3.2 Titanium and Titanium Alloys

Titanium and its alloys have been widely utilized as biomaterials, especially for prostheses, cardiovascular devices and fracture fixings, on account of its high biocompatibility, low density, low Young's modulus and superior corrosion resistance when compared with stainless steel. As an additional advantage, titanium has higher tendency to osseointegration, a relevant characteristic for long term implants [16].

Titanium reduced or inexistent reaction with the neighboring tissues around the implant results from passivation, formed by the titanium dioxide film (TiO_2), usually of nanometric thickness, on the metal surface [30, 31].

The disadvantage of commercially pure titanium (Ti-CP) is related to the poor wear resistance on usage, which renders it unsuitable for applications requiring high tension [30]. This is the reason why titanium has been utilized as the base element for forming alloys together with other chemical elements, such as aluminum, vanadium and iron aiming at improving the tensile forces (Ti-6Al-4V alloy).

In order to obtain titanium alloys of varied properties the alloys are modified by the addition of ligands and thermo mechanical processes. Titanium is an allotropic material having a compact hexagonal crystalline structure (α phase) up to 882 °C. Above this temperature the structure is altered into body centered cubic structure (β phase). Some elements, including Al, Sn and Zr stabilize the α phase while elements such as V, Mo, Nb and Mn stabilize the β phase. In this way, the alloy properties will depend on composition, relative proportions of α and β phases, thermal treatments and processing conditions. Titanium alloys of the α type have good corrosion resistance but limited mechanical resistance at low temperatures. On the contrary, the stabilized alloys of β phase have lower Young's modulus, which contributes to reduce the difference of this property between the biomaterial and the bone [31].

Among the different alloys involving titanium, the Ni-Ti alloy, called Nitinol, is being highlighted on account of its properties of shape memory, superelasticity, fatigue and torsion strength. The shape memory property refers to the ability of the material to regain the original shape after a deformation induced by temperature rise. The elastic behavior of Nitinol that enables deformation up to 20 times returning to the original dimensions after tension release. Due to these unique properties, the Ni-Ti alloy is utilized in orthodontic arches, guide-wires, stents, catheters, aneurism clips and orthopedic clamps [16, 31, 32].

3.3.3 Cobalt-Chrome-Based Alloys

Cobalt and chrome alloys for application as biomaterials are used in orthopedic prostheses for knee, shoulder and hip, fracture fixing devices, maxillofacial and dental implants [33, 34]. The wear resistance of the Co–Cr alloys is higher than that of stainless steels and of the titanium alloys. The disadvantages of these alloys are the low plasticity and the difficult machinability [32].

Analogously to stainless steel, corrosion resistance is due to formation of a protecting CrO_2 layer. Addition of small amounts of other elements such as iron, molybdenum and tungsten contributes to the improvement of properties at high temperatures and abrasion resistance. In this way, the two predominant alloys for use as biomaterials are the Co–Cr–Mo alloy and the Co–Cr–Ni–Mo alloy, commercially marketed as Vitallium. Other alloys approved for use include tungsten (Co–Cr–Ni–W) and iron (Co–Cr–Ni–W–Fe) [34].

3.3.4 Magnesium-Based Alloys

Magnesium alloys have attracted much attention in the field of orthopedic implant materials and tissue engineering, since the main alloy elements (Mg and Ca) can be tolerated by the body at relatively high levels. Alloys have mechanical properties compatible with the bone and are biodegradable. However, several drawbacks should be addressed before clinical applications, including hydrogen release (bubbles) resulting from corrosion and infection [16].

3.3.5 Tantalum

Tantalum is one of the refractory metals, among others which include niobium, molybdenum, tungsten and rhenium. Exception made to two of the platinum group metals (osmium and iridium), refractory metals have higher melting temperatures (>2000 °C) and the lowest vapor pressures of all. The use of niobium, molybdenum and tungsten for biomedical applications is restricted to alloys with stainless steels, cobalt alloys and titanium alloys. Radioactive rhenium is occasionally used in stents to prevent re-stenosis. Tantalum has a series of clinical applications on account of its excellent biocompatibility, flexibility and corrosion resistance [16].

3.3.6 Zirconium-Based Alloys

Zirconium is used mainly as an alloy element on account of its high corrosion resistance. By being refractory and having high oxygen affinity Zirconium is similar to titanium. Whenever zirconium is exposed to an oxygen-containing environment, a protecting oxide film is formed spontaneously on its surface, both under dry and wet conditions. Besides, the protecting film protects the base metal of chemical attack up to temperatures of 300 °C. As a result, zirconium is very resistant to corrosive attack of most mineral and organic acids, strong alkalis and salt solutions [16].

References

1. Sumita, M., Hanawa, T., Teoh, S.H.: Development of nitrogen-containing nickel-free. Mat. Sci. Eng. C. **24**(6–8), 753–760 (2004)
2. Poinern, G.E.J., Brundavanam, S., Fawcett, D.: Biomedical magnesium alloys: a review of material properties, surface modifications and potential as a biodegradable orthopaedic implant. Am. J. Biomed. Eng. **2**(6), 218–240 (2012)
3. Dee, K.C., Puleo, D.A., Bizios, R.: An introduction to tissue-biomate-rial interactions. Wiley, New Jersey (2002)
4. Park, J.B., Kim, Y.K.: Mettalic biomaterials. In: Park, J. B., Bronzino, J.D. (eds.) Biomaterials: Principles and Applications. CRC Press, Boca Raton (2002)
5. Ratner, B.D., Hoffman, A.S., Schoen, F.J., Lemons, J.E.: Biomaterials Science: An Introduction to Materials in Medicine, 3rd edn. Academic Press, Amsterdam (2013)
6. Blackwood, D.J.: Biomaterials: past successes and future problems. Corros. Rev. **21**(2–3), 97–124 (2003)
7. Geetha, M., Singh, A.K., Asokamani, R., Gogia, A.K.: Ti based biomaterials, the ultimate choice for orthopaedic implants—a review. Prog. Mater Sci. **54**, 397–425 (2009)
8. Duerig, T.W., Melton, K.N., Stockel, D., Wayman, C.M.: Engineering Aspects of Shape Memory Alloy. Butterworth-Heinemann, London (1990)
9. Staiger, M.P., Pietak, A.M., Huadmai, J., Dias, G.: Magnesium and its alloys as orthopedic biomaterials: a review. Biomaterials **27**(9), 1728–1734 (2006)
10. Heublein, B., Rohde, R., Kaese, V., Niemeyer, M., Hartung, W., Haverich, A.: Biocorrosion of magnesium alloys: a new principle in cardiovascular implant technology? Heart **89**(6), 651–656 (2003)
11. Wong, J.Y., Bronzino, J.D.: Biomaterials. CRC Press, New York (2007)
12. Food and Drug Administration.: Available at: http://www.fda.gov/MedicalDevices/ProductsandMedicalProcedures/DeviceApprovalsandClearances/default.htm (2011)

13. Mazzocca, A.D., DE Angelis, J.P., Caputo, A.E., Browner, B.D., Mast, J.W., Mendes, M.W.: Principles of internal fixation. In: Browner, B.D., Skeletal Trauma, W.B. (eds.) Saunders Company, Philadelphia (2008)
14. Okazaki, Y., Goth, E.: Metal release from stainless steel, CoCrMoNiFe and NiTi alloys in vascular implants. Corros. Sci. **50**(12), 3429–3438 (2008)
15. Hermawan, H. Introduction to Metals for Medical Devices. Available at: http://iomm.org.my/materials-mind/scientific-article-3-introduction-to-metals-for-medical-devices/. Accessed in January 2017
16. Chen, Q., Thouas, G.A.: Metallic implant biomaterials. Mat. Sci. Eng. R. **87**, 1–57 (2015)
17. Long, M., Rack, H.J.: Titanium alloys in total joint replacement—a materials science perspective. Biomaterials **19**, 1621–1639 (1998)
18. Niinomi, M.: Fatigue characteristics of mettalic biomaterials. Int. J. Fatigue **29**(6), 992–1000 (2007)
19. Sumita, M., Hanawa, T.: Failure processes in biometallic materials. Bioengineering, vol. 9, pp. 131–167. Elsevier Science Ltd., London (2003)
20. Shackelford, J.F.: Introduction to materials science for engineers. Pearson Pretice Hall, New Jersey (2008)
21. Manivasagam, G., Dhinasekaran, D., Rajamanickam, A.: Biomedical implants: corrosion and its prevention—a review. Recent Pat. Corros. Sci. **2**, 40–54 (2010)
22. Brockett, C.L., Harper, P., Williams, S., Isaac, G.H., Dwyer-Joyce, R.S., Jin, Z., Fisher, J.: The influence of clearance on friction, lubrication and squeaking in large diameter metal-on-metal hip replacements. J. Mater. Sci. Mater. Med. **19**(4), 1575–1579 (2008)
23. Nasab, M.B., Hassan, M.R.: Metallic biomaterials of knee and hip—a review. Trends Biomater. Artif. Organs. **24**, 69–82 (2010)
24. Subramanian, B., Ananthakumar, R., Kobayashi, A., Jayachandran, M.: Surface modification of 316L stainless steel with magnetron sputtered TiN/VN nanoscale multilayers for bio implant applications. J. Mater. Sci. Mater. Med. **23**, 329–338 (2012)
25. Parsapour, A., Khorasani, S.N., Fathi, M.H.J.: Effect of surface treatment and metallic coating on corrosion behavior and biocompatibility of surgical 316L stainless steel implant. Mater. Sci. Technol. **28**(2), 125–131 (2012)
26. Sammons, R.L.: Modifying biomaterial surfaces to optimise interactions with bone, In: Williams, R. (ed.) Surface Modification of Biomaterials—Methods, Analysis and Applications, pp. 365–391. Wood head Publishing, Oxford (2011)
27. Park, J., Lakes, R.S.: Biomaterials—An Introduction, 3rd edn. Springer, New York (2007)
28. International Agency For Research On Cancer. IARC—Monographs on the Evaluation of Carcinogenic Risks to Humans. Chrômium, Nickel and Welding. vol. 49, Lyon (1990)
29. Talha, M., Behera, C.K., Sinha, O.P.: A review on nickel-free nitrogen containing austenitic stainless steels for biomedical applications. Mat. Sci. Eng. C. **33**(7), 3563–3575 (2013)
30. Holzapfel, B.M., Reichert, J.C., Schantz, J.T., Gbureck, U., Rackwitz, L., Noth, U., Jakob, F., Rudert, M., Groll, J., Hutmacher, D.W.: How smart do biomaterials need to be? A translational science and clinical point of view. Adv. Drug Deliv. Rev. **65**(4), 581–603 (2013)
31. Liu, X., Chu, P.K., Ding, C.: Surface modification of titanium, titanium alloys, and related materials for biomedical applications. Mat. Sci. Eng. R. **47**(3–4), 49–121 (2004)
32. Hanawa, T.: Materials for metallic stents. Artif. Organs **12**(2), 73–79 (2009)
33. Marti, A.: Cobalt-base alloys used in bone surgery. Injury **4**, 18–21 (2000)
34. Paital, S.R., Dahotre, N.B.: Calcium phosphate coatings for bio-implant. Mat. Sci. Eng. R. **66** (1–3), 1–70 (2009)

Chapter 4
Ceramic Biomaterials

Since the bone tissue composition and characteristics are similar to those of ceramic materials, ceramics include a wide spectrum of compounds which played a relevant role in biomaterials development.

Ceramic materials are inorganic compounds, made up of metals and nonmetals linked by ionic and/or covalent bonds. In these bonds, electrons are located between the ions/atoms, forming crystalline structures. Therefore, ceramics tend to behave as low electrical and thermal conductivity [1]. The wide field of application in the medical area is due mainly to the crystallographic properties and to the superior chemical compatibility of ceramics with physiological medium and stiff tissues, such as bones and teeth [1, 2].

4.1 Obtention, Processing, and Application of Bioceramics

Raw materials utilized in the obtention of ceramic materials can be natural or synthesized from chemical reagents. For biomedical application ceramics, called Bioceramics by Hench, should be of high purity [3]. Ceramic materials are obtained according to the steps represented in Fig. 4.1.

The applications of these biomaterials encompass the most varied areas, such as diagnosis instruments, orthopedic prostheses, devices for dental and maxillofacial reconstruction, cardiac valves, artificial tracheae and bone replenishments (Fig. 4.2).

4.2 Properties of Bioceramics

Generally speaking, the density of ceramics is lower than that of most of metals and their alloys. These materials have good dimensional stability, are resistant to wear and to compression and stable in acidic media. However, the strong interatomic

V. dos Santos et al., *Engineering of Biomaterials*, Topics in Mining, Metallurgy and Materials Engineering, DOI 10.1007/978-3-319-58607-6_4

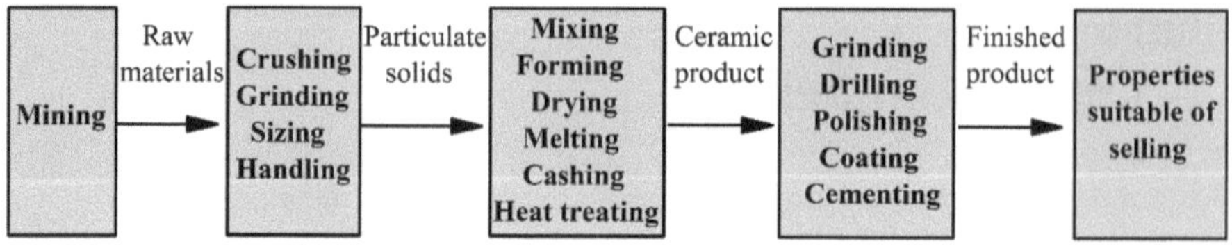

Fig. 4.1 Ceramic processing steps [3]

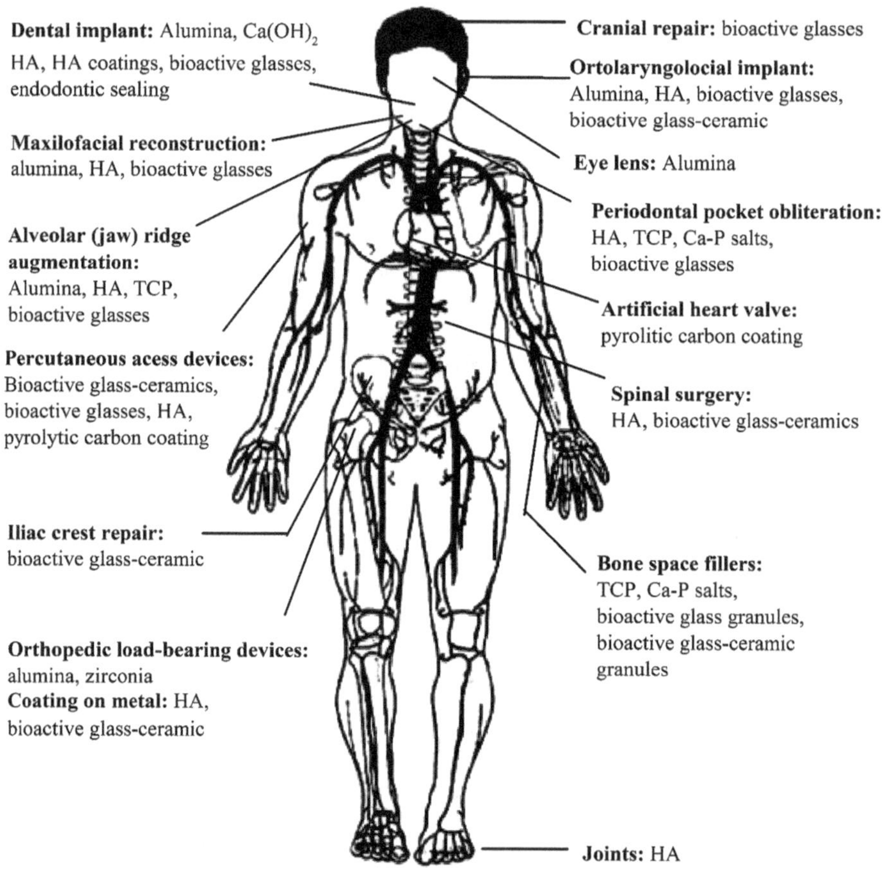

Fig. 4.2 Clinical application of ceramic biomaterials. Adapted [2]

bonds form tridimensional crystalline structures of high compaction degree, rendering them hard, brittle and susceptible to fracture, with low or no plastic deformation. Besides, they are very sensitive to flaws which may act as the onset of fractures and contribute to material breakdown during use. On account of these issues, ceramics are rarely recommended for applications in regions submitted to high tension and that demand support [2, 3].

Table 4.1 Types of bioceramics-tissue attachment and bioceramic classification [4]

Type of bioceramic	Type of attachment	Example
1.	Dense, nonporous, nearly inert ceramics attach by bone growth into surface irregularities by cementing the device into the tissues, or by press fitting into a defect (termed morphological fixation)	Al_2O_3 (single crystal and polycrystalline)
2.	For porous inert implants bone ingrowth occurs, which mechanically attaches the bone to the material (termed biological fixation)	Al_2O_3 (porous polycrystalline) Hydroxyapatite-coated porous metals
3.	Dense, nonporous, surface-reactive ceramics, glasses, and glass-ceramics attach directly by chemical bonding with the bone (termed bioactive fixation)	Bioactive glasses Bioactive glass-ceramics Hydroxyapatite
4.	Dense, nonporous (or porous), resorbable ceramics are designed to be slowly replaced by bone	Calcium sulfate (plaster or Paris) Tricalcium phosphate Calcium phosphate salts

The kinds of ceramic biomaterials are classed in accordance with Table 4.1 and the physical properties of alumina and partially stabilized zirconia are listed in Table 4.2 [4].

Table 4.2 Physical characteristics of alumina and partially stabilized zirconia (PSZ) bioceramics [4]

	High-alumina ceramics	ISO alumina standard 6474	PSZ	Cortical bone	Cancellous bone
Content (percent by weight)	$Al_2O_3 > 99.8$	$Al_2O_3 \geq 99.5$	$ZrO_2 > 97$		
Density (g/cm^3)	>3.93	$\geq$ 3.90	5.6–6.12	1.6–2.1	
Average grain size (μm)	3–6	<7	1		
Surface roughness R_a (μm)	0.02		0.008		
Hardness (Vickers), HV	2300	>2000	1300		
Compressive strength (MPa)	4500				2–12
Bending strength (MPa) (after testing in Ringer's solution)	550	400	1200	50–150	
Young's Modulus (GPa)	380		200	7–25	0.05–0.5
Fracture toughness, K_{IC} (MPa m$^{-1/2}$)	5–6		15	2–12	
Slow crack growth, n (unitless)	30–52		65		

Ceramic biomaterials are classed as bioinert, bioactive, and bioreabsorbable. Alumina and zirconia are bioinert while bioactive ceramics interact with the neighboring tissue, stimulating cure and the tissue system to respond to the material as this latter were a natural tissue. As examples of this class are highlighted hydroxyapatite, bioglasses, and vitroceramics. Tricalcium phosphate and gypsum are bioreabsorbable materials [3].

4.3 Types of Bioceramics

4.3.1 Alumina (Al_2O_3)

Alumina has a compact hexagonal crystalline structure, with characteristics of high hardness, compression, and abrasion resistance; it can be polished with high surface finishing. The strong ionic bonds and the high oxygen amount render it a chemically inert material, with high stability in physiologic and corrosive media [5].

The most widely utilized ceramic for implants is made up of high density and high purity (>99.5%) polycrystalline alumina (α-Al_2O_3). Tenacity and tensile strength and fatigue resistance of this kind of material is associated with the grain size and its purity. Small amounts of MgO (<0.5%) are frequently added aiming at inhibiting grain growth during sinterization to improve mechanical properties. Alumina of average grain size lower than 4 μm and with purity higher than 99.7% has good flexure strength and compression resistance. Grains of size in excess of 17 μm could diminish mechanical strength of alumina up to 20% [3, 5].

The main application of alumina is related to the manufacture of acetabula and femoral heads for hip arthroplasties. When these two pieces are polished together and utilized as a pair, the friction coefficient of the joint is reduced with time and the value tends to get close to that of normal articulation. Thus, the wear of the alumina–alumina surfaces is nearly 10 times lower than that of metal–polyethylene surfaces, for example. Other clinical applications of alumina include knee prostheses and elements for maxillofacial reconstruction, screws for bones, replacements for small bones of the middle ear, cornea prostheses, segmental replacements of bones, and dental implants [3].

The mechanical strength of monocrystalline alumina (sapphire) is nearly three times higher than that of polycrystalline alumina, good esthetics and possibility of obtention of devices of different sizes and shapes. Such material had wide utilization in the manufacture of dental prostheses and crowns. However, its use was reduced due to its low impact resistance [6]. Currently, monocrystalline alumina is employed as bracket in orthodontic devices on account of its better esthetics and highly polished surface. For this purpose, however, this material may present some drawbacks such as the possibility of fracture and high attrition during the sliding mechanics, which can produce some discomfort for the patient [7].

4.3.2 Zirconia (ZrO_2)

Zirconia belongs to the group of inert ceramics and has a polymorphic structure with three different forms of crystal: monoclinic (M), cubic (C), and tetragonal (T). The monoclinic structure is observed at temperatures up to 1170 °C. Above this, the transformation to the tetragonal occurs and at 2370 °C zirconia takes the cubic phase [8]. During cooling from the processing temperature on, the tetragonal phase turns into the monoclinic phase together with volume expansion (3–4%) which causes inner tensions in the material microstructure, producing cracks that render it extremely fragile. Thus, mechanical and refractory properties of neat zirconia are jeopardized, limiting its applications.

Aiming at increasing the mechanical strength and tenacity, the tetragonal and cubic crystalline phases can be stabilized at low temperatures by the use of additives, such as the magnesium, cerium, yttrium, and calcium oxides. According to the additives concentration, this procedure can originate tetragonal polycrystalline zirconia (TPZ), fully stabilized zirconia (FSZ, normally in the cubic phase) and partially stabilized zirconia (PSZ) where fine metastable tetragonal particles are dispersed into a cubic matrix [9, 10]. Among the different modified forms, the yttrium-stabilized tetragonal polycrystalline zirconia (Y-TZP) is highlighted for having very fine grains and low porosity. These factors make it possible, the obtention of a material of high tensile strength, tenacity and resistance to erosive wear, which can be successively utilized in applications submitted to mechanical tensions [9]. As compared with alumina, this ceramic has higher strength, lower hardness, and lower elastic modulus. The main applications of zirconia are as an alternative material to alumina in the manufacture of femoral heads for hip prostheses, knee, and shoulder prostheses and dental materials [10, 11]. There is also growing interest in the combined utilization of zirconia and alumina aiming at obtaining devices of mechanical and degradation properties adjusted to the desired application [3].

4.3.3 Calcium Phosphate Ceramics

Calcium phosphate ceramics have high potential for application as biomaterial on account of their chemical and structural similarity with biological apatite, present in huge amounts in bones and teeth mineral phase. These materials have excellent biocompatibility and bioactive behavior, making it possible high levels of bone integration and bone conduction [3, 12].

Calcium phosphates have been widely studied and employed for applications encompassing all of the skeletal system, such as skull-maxillofacial and treatment of bone defects reconstructions. Still, calcium phosphate porous ceramics can act as useful supports for the release of different compounds incorporated in them, such as hormones [13], vaccines [14], antibiotics [15], and anticancer agents, including radioactive compounds [16] and cisplatin [17, 18]. The main limitations to the use of calcium phosphate stem from the fact that they are very brittle and have low fatigue resistance. That is why dense or porous coatings of these ceramics are frequently applied to supporting metallic implants in order to enable biological attachment or osseointegration.

Calcium phosphates are made up of phosphoric or orthophosphoric acid salts and can be synthesized by precipitation from Ca^{2+} and PO_4^{3-} containing solutions under alkaline or acidic conditions. The molar ratio between the calcium and phosphorous atoms (Ca/P) varies between 0.5 and 2.0 and is usually utilized as a tool to class the different calcium phosphates. Compounds of higher Ca/P ratio are less soluble under neutral conditions and reduced degradation rate [19, 20].

Among the most widely spread calcium phosphates are hydroxyapatite, $Ca_{10}(PO_4)_6(OH)_2$ and tricalcium phosphate under the polymorphic α and β $Ca_3(PO_4)_2$ forms the surfaces which favor protein absorption and have high bone inductive potential.

Hydroxyapatite (HP) is one of the main components of bone minerals, enamel, and dentine and is also present in urinary and dental calculi [20]. As a biomaterial, it has the advantages of quick bone adaptation, no formation of fibrous tissue, reduced crystallization time, and intimate implant/tissue adhesion. The limitation of this compound is related to its low biodegradation, which occurs by cell mechanisms gradually after 4–5 years of implantation. This behavior can be attributed to the 1.67 Ca/P molar ratio that renders HP practically insoluble in neutral media.

Tricalcium phosphates (TCP) which have Ca/P of 1.5, are not stable in aqueous solutions and in humid environments, being reabsorbed between 6 and 15 weeks after the implant, depending on some factors such as porosity, crystallinity, chemical purity, and biomaterial surface roughness [3, 21]. The allotropic forms α and β-TCP exhibit the same capacity of bone conduction, however the α TCP phase is of higher bioactivity, this fact being attributed to the structural arrangement of this phase, which makes it possible higher amounts of Ca^{2+} and PO_4^{3} to be exchanged with the biological medium [20].

Both described calcium phosphates are under study to be used as scaffolds in the area of tissue engineering however, as TCP degrades more rapidly than HA (it undergoes simultaneously the action of cellular and chemical mechanisms) the prediction and control of its degradation rate is more difficult. In this way, the use of TCP together with HA has been a viable alternative to increase HA reabsorption rate. In these cases, the velocity of dissolution of the HA/TCP mixture is controlled by the amount of TCP utilized [20].

4.3.4 Calcium Phosphate Cements (CPC)

These materials (CPC) are biodegradable and multicomponents, made up of an inorganic solid phase and a liquid phase, which, upon being admixed, form a paste that stiffens spontaneously at ambient or corporeal temperature as a result of the precipitation of one or several calcium phosphates. During the precipitation reaction, CaP crystals grow and intertwine, providing in this way the mechanical stiffness to the cement [22]. The inorganic phase can be made up by one or more calcium phosphates and the liquid phase is made up of water or aqueous solutions. Several characteristics render the calcium phosphates cements attractive for utilization as bone grafts and replacements, such as ease in manipulation and non-toxicity, the possibility of being injected, which renders surgical processes less invasive, and the ability to provide solidification in situ, without appreciable heat generation and good adjustment to the implant site, even at geometrically complex defects, assuring better contact of tissue and biomaterial. Besides, there is the possibility of incorporation into these materials of growth factors in order to stimulate specific biological reactions and of drugs for the controlled release at predetermined locations of the skeletal system [23–25].

Among the disadvantages of this material are the low mechanical strength as compared with the normal bone and the fact of being devoid of microporosity, which hinders cellular growth within it.

4.3.5 Bioglasses and Vitroceramics

The use of bioactive glasses started with the innovative development of Bioglass® 45S5 by Larry Hench in 1969. It is made up of a quaternary system of the SiO_2–CaO–Na_2O–P_2O_5 kind, and this is still considered the base model for bioglasses, where 45% by mass is made up by SiO_2 and the CaO and P_2O_5 ratio should be 5:1 for the interfacial bond to the bone to occur [3, 4, 26]. This composition has excellent interaction properties with living tissues and bone induction. Formulations having from 52 to 60% by mass of SiO_2 have slower bonding rates with the bone tissue. Above 60% SiO_2 there is no bond formation with the tissue and the material acquires the bioinert behavior [27].

When implanted in the body, at the surface of this material a carbonated, biologically active hydroxyapatite layer is formed, which is responsible for the strong interfacial bond to the bone tissue [19, 27]. The force of interfacial adhesion resists to substantial mechanical efforts and, in many cases, is stronger than the implant material cohesion force or that of the tissue [3]. Bioglass® can also have interaction with the conjunctive tissue, provided the interface is motionless [27]. More recently, it was observed that ionic dissolution of bioglass products (Si, Ca, P) stimulate the expression of several genes of osteoblast cells and angiogenesis in vitro and in vivo [21].

The formation of the hydroxyapatite layer occurs by a chemical mechanism involving five distinct phases (Fig. 4.3). In the first step, there is a quick Na^+ ions exchange of the glass surface with H^+ and H_3O^+ solution ions. In the second step, the glass soluble silica (SiO_2) is released as $Si(OH)_4$ towards the solution, as a result of siloxane bonds (Si–O–Si) breakage and formation of silinol (Si–OH) groups at the interface. The third step is characterized by polycondensation of the silinol

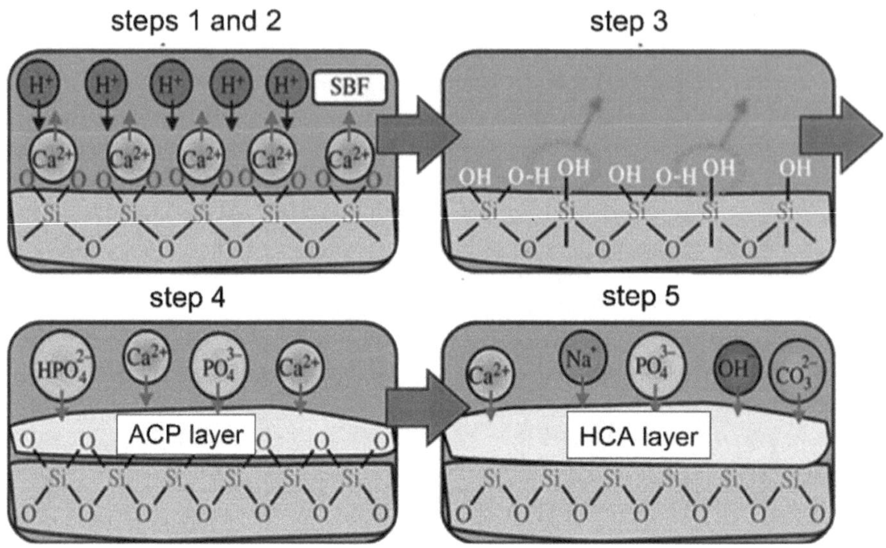

Fig. 4.3 Mechanism of hydroxyapatite layer formation [27]

groups forming a silica-rich porous layer at the material surface, already deficient in alkaline and alkaline earth cations. During the next step, Ca^{2+} ions and $(PO_4)^{3-}$ groups migrate from the surface forming a $CaO–P_2O_6$, rich film which grows in an amorphous way by additionally incorporating soluble calcium and phosphates of the physiological solution. In the last step, the amorphous film is crystallized by incorporating OH and CO_3^{2-} ions present in solution, yielding the carbonated hydroxyapatite layer. The size of crystals formed at the surface of the bioactive glass tends to be in the nanometric scale, equivalent to the bone crystalline phase [27, 28].

The ability of bioglasses in stimulating bone growth exceeds that of the hydroxyapatite-based implants. The bioactivity index, related to the period of time so that more than 50% of the biomaterial surface is linked to the tissue cells is of 12.5 for Bioglass® 45S5 while that of hydroxyapatite is 3.1 [29]. In this way, while Bioglass® 45S5 would take nearly 8 days for 50% of its surface to be linked to the tissue cells, HA would need nearly 32 days, if utilized under the same conditions [27].

The most common applications for bioactive glasses include bone repair and regeneration, including orthopedics, periodontics, maxillofacial reconstruction, backbone surgery and otorhinolaryngologistic reconstructions [28].

The limitations of this compound stem from the poor mechanical resistance, mainly the fracture strength, and the restricted machinability [27]. In search of improving these properties, the development of thermal treatments was sought for crystals nucleation and growth in bioactive glasses, which originated vitroceramics. Since then, various systems were obtained such as Ceravital ($Na_2O–K_2O–MgO–CaO–SiO_2–P_2O_5$), Bioverit I ($SiO_2–Al_2O_3–MgO–CaO–P_2O_5$), and A-W Cerabone

($MgO–CaO–SiO–P_2O_5–CaF_2$) [27, 30]. The increased crystallinity of the obtained materials modifies their physical and chemical properties, as well as tends to reduce their bioactivity.

Production of bioceramics of controlled microstructure based on compositions similar to that of Bioglass® 45S5 has been studied aiming at combining the superior mechanical properties of vitroceramics and the high bioglasses bioactivity. This new material, called Biosilicato®, of crystallinity close to 100%, exhibits high bioactivity and its Young's modulus is closer to that of the cortical bone. As a particulate, this material does not have cutting edges and its higher potential use would be in the treatment of dentin hypersensitivity. In the presence of mouth fluids, when deposited within the dental tubules, this material can onset the HA formation process, resulting in its occlusion by means of a chemical bond with the material [27].

References

1. Shackelford, J.F.: Introduction to Materials Science for Engineers. Pearson Pretice Hall, New Jersey (2008)
2. Park, J., Lakes, R.S.: Biomaterials: An Introduction, 3rd edn. Springer, New York (2007)
3. Ratner, B.D., Hoffman, A.S., Schoen, F.J., Lemons, J.E.: Biomaterials Science: An Introduction to Materials in Medicine, 3rd edn. Academic Press, Amsterdam (2013)
4. Hench, L.L.: Bioceramic: from concept to clinic. J. Am. Cer. Soc. **74**(7), 1487–1510 (1991)
5. Pezzotti, G., Yamamoto, K.: Artificial hip joints: the biomaterials challenge. J. Mech. Behav. Biomed. Mater. **31**, 3–20 (2014)
6. Haubenreich, J.E., Robinson, F.G., West, K.P., Frazer, R.Q.: Did we push dental ceramics too far? A brief history of ceramic dental implants. J. Long-Term Eff. Med. Implants. **15**(6), 617–628 (2005)
7. Pimentel, R.F., Oliveira, R.S.M.F., Chaves, M.G.A.M., Elias, C.N., Gravina, M.A.: Evaluation of the friction force generated by monocristalyne and policristalyne ceramic brackets in sliding mechanics. Dental Press J. Orthod. **18**, 121–127 (2013)
8. Afzal, A.: Implantable zirconia bioceramics for bone repair and replacement: a chronological review. Mater. Express. **4**, 1–12 (2014)
9. Yoshimura, H.N., Molisani, A.L., Narita, N.E., Gonçalves, M.P., Campos, M.F.: Zircônia parcialmente estabilizada de baixo custo produzida por meio de mistura de pós com aditivos do sistema $MgO–Y_2O_3CaO$. Cerâmica. **53**, 116–132 (2007)
10. Piconi, C., Maccauro, G.: Zirconia as a ceramic biomaterial. Biomaterials **20**, 1–25 (1999)
11. Thamaraiselvi, T.V., Rajeswari, S.: Biological evaluation of bioceramic materials—a review trends. Trends Biomater. Artif. Organs. **18**, 9–17 (2004)
12. Dorozhkin, S.V.: Bioceramics of calcium orthophosphates. Biomaterials **31**, 1465–1485 (2010)
13. Paul, W., Sharma, C.P.: Porous hydroxyapatite nanoparticles for intestinal delivery of insulin. Trends Biomater. Artif. Organs. **25**, 91–94 (2011)
14. Sahdev, P., Podaralla, S., Kaushik, R.S., Perumal, O.: Calcium phosphate nanoparticles for transcutaneous vaccine delivery. J. Biomed. Nanotechnol. **9**, 132–141 (2013)
15. Kim, H.W., Knowles, J.C., Kim, H.E.: Hydroxyapatite porous scaffold engineered with biological polymer hybrid coating for antibiotic Vancomycin release. J. Mater. Sci. Mater. Med. **16**(3), 189–195 (2005)

16. Lacerda, K.A., Lameiras, F.S., Silva, V.V.: Avaliação da biodegradação de matrizes porosas à base de hidroxiapatita para aplicação como fontes radioativas em braquiterapia. Quim. Nova **32**(5), 1216–1221 (2009)
17. Netz, D.J.A., Sepulveda, P., Pandolfelli, V.C., Spadaro, A.C.C., Alencastre, J.B., Bentley, M. V.L.B., Marchetti, J.M.: Potential use of gelcasting hydroxyapatite porous ceramic as an implantable drug delivery system. Int. J. Pharm. **213**, 117–125 (2001)
18. Barroug, A., Kuhn, L.T., Gerstenfeld, L.C., Glimcher, M.J.: Interactions of cisplatin with calcium phosphate nanoparticles: in vitro controlled adsorption and release. J. Orthop. Res. **22**(4), 703–708 (2004)
19. Best, S.M., Porter, A.E., Huang, J.: Bioceramics: past, present and for the future. J. Eur. Ceram. Soc. **28**(7), 1319–1327 (2008)
20. Guastaldi, A.C., Aparecida, A.H.: Fosfatos de cálcio de interesse biológico: importância como biomateriais, propriedades e métodos de obtenção de recobrimentos Quim. Nova. **33**(6), 1352–1358 (2010)
21. Hoppe, A., Güldal, N.S., Boccaccini, A.R.: A review of the biological response to ionic dissolution products from bioactive glasses and glass-ceramics. Biomaterials **32**(11), 2757–2774 (2011)
22. Bohner, M.: Calcium orthophosphates in medicine: from ceramics to calcium phosphate cements. Injury **4**, 37–47 (2000)
23. Ginebra, M.P., Traykova, T., Planell, J.A.: Calcium phosphate cements as bone drug delivery systems: a review. J. Control. Release. **113**(2), 102–110 (2006)
24. Ambard, A.J.: Calcium phosphate cement: review of mechanical and biological properties. J. Prosthodont. **15**(5), 321–328 (2006)
25. Zhang, J., Liu, W., Schnitzler, V., Tancret, F., Bouler, J.M.: Calcium phosphate cements for bone substitution: chemistry, handling and mechanical properties. Acta Biomater. **10**(3), 1035–1049 (2014)
26. Jones, J.R.: Review of bioactive glass: from Hench to hybrids. Acta Biomater. **9**(1), 4457–4486 (2013)
27. Siqueira, R.L., Zanotto, E.D.: Biosilicato®: histórico de uma vitrocerâmica brasileira de elevada bioatividade. Quim. Nova **34**(7), 1231–1241 (2011)
28. Hench, L.L., Roki, N., Fenn, M.B.: Bioactive glasses: importance of structure and properties in bone regeneration. J. Mol. Struct. **1073**, 24–30 (2014)
29. Hench, L.L.: Bioceramics: from concept to clinic. J. Am. Cer. Soc. **74**, 1487–1310 (1991)
30. Mundstock, K.B., Oliveira, A.P.N., Hotza, D., Rogero, S.O.: Processamento e caracterização de espumas vitrocerâmicas do sistema SNCP (SiO_2–Na_2O–CaO–P_2O_5). Quim. Nova **33**(3), 598–602 (2010)

Chapter 5
Polymeric Biomaterials

Currently, polymers represent the largest class of materials utilized in medicine, being widely employed in several applications as biomaterials, such as orthopedics, dentistry, hard and soft tissue replacements, cardiovascular devices, and others [1].

The widespread use of polymeric biomaterials is mainly due to their physical chemical properties, structural mobility, and ease of processing and shaping, which enable to confer to these materials characteristics suitable for each specific application [2, 3]. As disadvantages, the polymeric materials show poor mechanical properties, if compared with metals and ceramics, such as time-depending degradation as well as exposure conditions, besides hard properties maintenance after sterilization. This latter disadvantage, sterilization, will be addressed in Chap. 7 of this book.

5.1 Fundamental Concepts of Polymers

Polymers are macromolecules formed from smaller structural units (the monomers). Monomers are low molar weight molecules which, based on polymerization reactions, can produce macromolecules having repeating units called unit mer linked together. Polymers are basically made up of carbon and hydrogen linked by covalent bonds, the properties and applications being completely altered by the inclusion of oxygen, chlorine or fluorine, or sulfur and/or nitrogen in the repeating unit. The chemical structure of the polymeric materials, due to the presence of chemical elements of different electro negativities and/or spatial geometry of the chemical bonds makes that polymers can be hydrophilic or hydrophobic, and this characteristic also influences the response of this kind of material as biomaterial. The kind of chemical elements of the repeating unit and the strength of the chemical bond between them is the basis for the difference of polymeric biomaterials relative to metals and ceramics.

V. dos Santos et al., *Engineering of Biomaterials*, Topics in Mining, Metallurgy and Materials Engineering, DOI 10.1007/978-3-319-58607-6_5

In order to enable the better understanding of polymeric materials suitable for use as a biomaterial, some concepts and classifications should be worked out in this chapter.

The physical, chemical, thermal, rheological, and mechanical behavior among other characteristics of polymeric materials is influenced by their synthesis or polymerization reaction. Polymers can be obtained from natural sources such as natural rubber (NR), polyhydroxybutirate, chitosan collagen, proteins, sugar cane, or they can be of synthetic origin such as the petroleum or natural gas-based polymers, among other sources, this latter being a source of numerous polymers.

From natural sources, due to the complexity of media from which the polymers are extracted, and the difference among biological species, the purification of this kind of polymer can be relatively complex.

From synthetic processes, based on monomers and according to Carothers, the kind of polymerization reaction can be by addition and by condensation. As for the polymerization mechanism, according to Flory, polymerization occurs by chain growth and step growth [4]. These differences in polymerization make it possible to produce different characteristics and properties for the obtained polymers. Besides the different polymerization reactions, polymers can be produced by different methodologies for performing polymerization reactions, the so-called physical arrangements, such as: mass, solution, suspension, and emulsion polymerization [5].

Addition polymerization produces polymers such as polyethylene, polypropylene, polystyrene, polytetrafluoroethylene, poly(vinyl chloride), polyacrylonitrile, poly (methyl methacrylate), besides copolymers. Condensation polymerization produces high performance polymers, which bear properties and costs differentiated from the remaining polymers, such as polysulfones, poly(ether-ether-ketone) besides polymers such as polyurethane, poly(ethylene terephthalate), poly (butylene terephthalate), polycarbonate, polyamides above polyamide-6, and all kinds of resins used after cross-linking for obtaining composites (polyester resin, urea-formaldehyde resin, phenol-formaldehyde resin, vinyl resin and epoxy resin).

A further classification which differentiates polymeric materials is related to their solubility and fusibility, in which polymers can be classified as thermoplastics and thermosetting. In the first one, polymers melt by heating and solidify by cooling and may be recycled. In the second one, once cross-links are formed by temperature, catalysts, and additives, the same become insoluble and infusible.

Polymer blend is defined as a system originating from the physical admixture of two or more polymers, without a high degree of chemical reaction among them [6]. This is different from composites that according to the ASTM D3878-15 [7] Method refer to a substance consisting of two or more materials, insoluble one in the other, combined aiming at forming a useful engineering material, which possesses certain properties absent from each constituent taken separately. Composites employed in biomaterials will be addressed in Chap. 6 of this book.

Number average molecular weight (Mn) and weight average molecular weight (Mw) of polymeric materials can influence the properties and behavior of the same regarding their use.

Another characteristic of polymeric materials which can influence its behavior as biomaterial is the index of crystallinity (Xc). Polymeric materials can be semicrystalline or amorphous. The index of crystallinity, in %, influences thermal, chemical, rheological, mechanical, and biological properties, and consequently, influences the polymeric material behavior as biomaterial.

5.1.1 Synthetic Polymers Used as Biomaterials

Table 5.1 lists the main synthetic polymers used as biomaterials, their properties, and limitations.

5.1.2 Concepts of Degradation, Biodegradation, Bioabsorption and Bioreabsorption

Polymers applied in medicine besides being classified relative to the origin, as natural or synthetic, are also classified relative to the behavior exhibited when exposed to the corporeal environment. They can be stable, biodegradable, or bioreabsorbable [3].

The concepts of degradation, biodegradation, bioabsorption, and bioreabsorption can have several meanings, therefore it is necessary to differentiate them and define them in the way they will be used in this book.

According to DePaoli [10], the phenomena that lead to the degradation of a polymeric material can be combined, for example: exposure to an aggressive environment with mechanical demand, or during the production of a biomaterial, there are thermal and mechanical effects. Standardized definitions for biodegradation were also set forth in agreement with the ISO 472:13 norm [11], ASTMD6004-04:11 [12], ASTM 883:12 [13], ASTM D20.96 [14].

The Consensus Conference of the European Society for Biomaterials refers to biodegradation only when the main degradation process is biotic, that is, it occurs by the action of a biological agent (bacteria, fungi and algae). Thus, the degradation of poly (lactic acid) (PLA) cannot be described as biodegradation, since the process which precedes biodegradation is hydrolysis (predominantly) [15]. According to Proikakis et al. [16], the hydrolysis process is ruled by four basic parameters: the velocity constant, the amount of absorbed water, the diffusion coefficient of the chain fragments within the polymer, and the solubility of the degradation products. This process can further be affected by such parameters as, structure, molar mass, and its distribution and crystallinity, besides the shape of its test specimens, thermal, and mechanical history (including processing) [17].

Hydrolytic degradation of a solid polymer matrix can occur by two alternative processes [16]: (1) surface/core or heterogeneous erosion or (2) mass erosion (matrix core) or homogeneous erosion. When the process is heterogeneous,

Table 5.1 Synthetic polymers used as biomaterials [8, 9]

Polymer (Initials)	Properties	Limitation
Ultra High Molecular Weight Polyethylene (UHMWPE)	Mn = 2.000,000–5.000,000 g/mol Xc = 45% Abrasion Resistance superior to that of the other thermoplastics, inferior only to alumina, Good corrosion resistance, High resistance to cyclic fatigue, High resistance to tensile fracture, High chemical resistance, High hardness, Low friction coefficient, Resistant to chemicals: acids, alkalis, solvents, fuels, detergents and oxidants, Resistant to δ radiation under controlled conditions, Resistant to the action of ethylene oxide, Products obtained: in the shape of plates, bars, rods, tubes, or slabs for further finishing by machining, Due to its resistance to scission can be processed without additives or stabilizers	Subject to degradation by UV radiation and oxygen, Practically infusible, therefore not processable by conventional methods, Compression Molding or variations with pressing and extrusion by piston, Ram, Micro particles formation by wear of parts, followed by inflammation process and loss and deterioration of neighboring tissues, mainly at the bone at which it is anchored leading to pain, loss of function or need of replacement
High Density Polyethylene (HDPE)	Xc (80–90%) Mn = 100,000 g/mol Young's modulus = 1.2 GPa Chemical resistance, Resistant to oils and greases, Easy processing and shaping Low cost	Does not resist to certain kinds of sterilization (δ radiation, autoclave)
Polypropylene (PP)	Xc (60–70%) Mn = 10^4–10^5 g/mol Young's modulus = 1.5 GPa High stiffness, Good chemical resistance High mechanical resistance (31 MPa) Resistance to embrittlement superior to PE Nontoxic Easy processing and shaping Low cost	Does not resist to certain kinds of sterilization (δ radiation, autoclave)

(continued)

Table 5.1 (continued)

Polymer (Initials)	Properties	Limitation
Poly(vinyl chloride) (PVC)	Xc (5–15%) Mn = 10^4–10^5 g/mol Young's modulus = 3 GPa Utilized as tubes for biomedical applications, PVC is used with plasticizers in order to enable its processing, Low cost	Plasticizers added to PVC are highly toxic and can be extracted by the body Plasticizers for medium and long-term applications can cause drawbacks Does not resist to certain kinds of sterilization (δ radiation, autoclave)
Polytetrafluoro ethylene (PTFE)	Xc = 95% Mn = 10^5–10^6 g/mol Young's modulus = 0.5 GPa Thermal and chemically stable, Highly hydrophobic and excellent lubricity, In micro porous form utilized as vascular suture	Does not resist to certain kinds of sterilization and undergoes higher wear as compared with UHMWPE Processing as hard as that of UHMWPE
Poly(methyl methacrylate) (PMMA)	Xc = amorphous Mn = 10^5–10^6 Young's modulus = 2.9 GPa Vitreous (amorphous), Transparent, Good transmittance, Good tenacity, Hydrophobic, Can assume different viscosity conditions from stiff to gel	As a bone cement in prostheses can lead to fibrosis, pain and need to implant withdrawing Does not resist to certain kinds of solvents
Polycarbonate (PC)	Vitreous (amorphous) Mn = 3×10^4 g/mol Young's modulus = 2.8 GPa Transparent, High thermal resistance, High mechanical resistance (72 Mpa) High chemical resistance, In admixture with other polymers can be used in applications in contact with tissues and blood It replaces glass and sometimes PVC which does not meet more stringent technical requirements	Does not resist to certain kinds of solvents Combination of tensile and impact resistance, usually exhibits antagonistic behavioral properties
Polyamide 6.6 (PA)	Xc = variable Mn = 2×10^4 g/mol Young's modulus = 2.8 GPa Hygroscopic, water acts as plasticizer and can attack the amorphous region	Enzymes can attack the amide group and aid in the polymer hydrolysis

(continued)

Table 5.1 (continued)

Polymer (Initials)	Properties	Limitation
Polyurethane (PU)	Xc and Mn = Depends on the synthesis Young's modulus = variable Tensile Strength = variable Resistance to fatigue and degradation in biological environments Produced from castor bean oil as a replacement to Polyol, biodegradable	Does not resist to certain kinds of sterilization. Toxicity of the synthesis monomers
Poly(dimethyl siloxane) (PDMS) Silicone	Xc = variable Mn = 10^5–10^6 g/mol Thermostability, High folding resistance, Low bacterial adhesion, Extremely high biocompatibility, Generally hydrophobic, Highly compressible, High corrosion resistance, Low chemical reactivity Can be produced as liquid, gel, elastomeric and stiff	Does not resist to certain kinds of sterilization. Drainage Silicone implants do not last forever (10 or more years), The breast implant can impair the mammography, The scar tissue formed around the implant can press it, change in breast shape

Xc = crystallinity, Mn = molecular weight

polymer degradation occurs at different rates at the surface and on the inside owing to the difference in water absorption in these regions, it being quicker at the surface than in the interior or quicker in the interior than at the surface. For a homogeneous process, the matrix degrades slowly and water absorption by the system is quicker than polymer degradation. Thus, the system is quickly hydrated and polymer chains are cleaved along the material [16].

According to Barbanti, Zavaglia and Duek [18], the degradation process of poly (α-hydroxyacids) in body fluids can be described as a sequence of events. At first, there is degradation of the material, followed by ester linkages hydrolysis (which yields oligomers or monomers), then degradation proceeds through a biologically active process, performed by enzymes or by a passive hydrolytic cleavage process. This step is evidenced by reduced weight average molecular weight and loss of mechanical properties.

Bioreabsorption by living beings body occurs when products and by-products generated by degradation exhibit characteristics of the organic metabolites, specially the Krebs cycle acids. For PLA reabsorption and metabolization in vivo occur because of lactic acid obtention as a product of its degradation and in the body lactic acid is converted into pyruvic acid that in the presence of acetyl coenzyme A releases carbon dioxide (CO_2) and decomposes into citrate. On its turn, the citrate is inserted in the citric acid cycle, also known as Krebs cycle and eventually results in CO_2 and water (H_2O), enabling it to be discarded by urine and breathing [18].

Heller [19] suggests that a polymer is considered bioerodible when it has been insoluble in water and converted, under physiological conditions, into water soluble materials, without any concern with the specific mechanism involved in the erosion process. For Ratner [1], bioerosion includes physical processes such as dissolution, swelling, and deformation. The mere solubilization of the polymer, resulting from pH variations, can lead it to erosion, however, bioerosion includes chemical processes such as structural disintegration, mass loss, and possible function loss. These changes in the characteristics of polymeric materials integrate the concept of degradation explained in this chapter. The expression bio in bioerosion indicates that erosion occurred under physiological conditions or by action of a biological agent.

In the last decades, biodegradable and bioreabsorbable polymers of synthetic origin, such as PLA, poly (glycolic acid) (PGA), poly (lactic acid-co-glycolic acid) (PLGA), poly(ε-caprolactone) (PCL) and their copolymers were extensively studied for pharmaceutical and medical applications [20]. The interest in this class of materials is mainly due to its behavior in biological media. For example, the use of bioreabsorbable implants is advantageous relative to conventional metallic implants, as the implant will gradually degrade in the body and lead to products which will be reabsorbed and eliminated by the metabolic route there will be no need of a second surgery for implant removal, as is the case with the metallic ones, besides, the bioreabsorbable implant will provide a reduction in built up tension and consequently patient pain relief [20, 21].

Bioabsorption and bioreabsorption are used to indicate that the polymer or its degradation products are removed by cell activity (for example, phagocytosis).

Degradable polymers exhibit more stringent requirements in terms of biocompatibility than the nondegradable materials. Biocompatibility is understood, according to Oréfice [3] described in Chap. 2.

Besides the potential problems of toxic contaminants (residual monomers, stabilizers, initiators, emulsifiers, etc.) used in the synthesis and modification of properties, the toxic potential of the polymer materials degradation products, which limits the amount of materials to be employed as biomaterials, should be taken into consideration.

There are several biopolymers utilized for obtaining materials for biomedical applications, proteins (such as collagen, elastin, and silk fibroin), and polysaccharides (such as chitosan, alginate, xanthan gum, hyaluronic acid, and pectin) being highlighted [22, 23]. Applications for regenerative medicine include wound treatment and timed release drugs, among others, attributed to the biodegradability and biocompatibility characteristics as well as similarity with the extracellular matrix and for inducing and stimulating the wound cicatrization process [24, 25].

According to Kim and Kim [26] in order that a synthetic polymer may be degradable, it is necessary that it could be used as a nutrient for microorganisms under conditions for these microorganisms to proliferate. Microorganisms secrete enzymes and these are in charge of the material degradation.

A few characteristics of polymeric materials could favor biodegradation and therefore make it possible different applications of these as biomaterials. These are: hydrophilicity, in a general way, enzymatic hydrolysis of a certain polymer will depend on the hydrophilicity of the polymer chain. Since the microorganism's attack should always occur at the polymer surface, the onset of the hydrolysis degradation could be made easier by increased superficial hydrophilicity of the polymer. An additional variable is the degree of crystallinity, which will affect water diffusion through the polymer superficial layers, the lower it is, the better for biodegradation and the worse for mechanical properties. Besides, enzymatic attack is impaired at stiff segment regions [26]. The presence of certain functional groups such carbonyls, carboxyls, hydroxyls, branched chains, and low molar mass can favor the biodegradation process.

5.1.3 Main Polymers Biodegradable, Bioreabsorbable, Bioerodible Utilized as Biomaterials

Table 5.2 lists the main polymers utilized as biomaterials, their properties, and limitations.

The hydrogels category of polymeric materials is also to be highlighted whenever it relates to biomaterials.

5.2 Polymeric Hydrogels

Hydrogels are materials possessing as main characteristics the ability of absorbtion and retaining water into their structure (20–100% water relative to the total mass), without dissolution of the material. This kind of polymeric material by means of cross-linking forms a hydrophilic tridimensional network among chains. Hydrogen bonds, bio-recognition interactions, hydrophobic interactions, polymer crystallites, and physical entanglements of individual chains or a combination of two or more of the above interactions can influence water absorption ability. Ionic character in the structure also influences since repulsion is important for promoting polymer swelling in aqueous fluids [27].

Water absorption mechanism by a dry hydrogel starts by the hydration of the hydrophilic and polar groups having as consequence the expansion of the network exposing the hydrophobic groups which can also interact, by van der Waals forces, with water molecules. Hydrogels' volume expansion is limited by the cross-linking degree and polymeric chain entanglement. Hydrogels can be classified by their method of preparation and ionic charge. Based on the method of preparation they can be: homopolymers (cross-linked chain polymers of one single monomer kind),

Table 5.2 Biodegradable, bioreabsorbable, bioerodible polymers utilized as biomaterials [1, 3, 9]

Polymer (Initial)	Properties	Limitation	
Poly(lactic acid) (PLA)	Density = 1.21–1.25 g/cm^3 Tensile strength = 21–60 MPa Young's modulus = 0.35–3.5 GPa D-PLA-semicrystalline L-PLA-semicrystalline D,L-PLA-amorphous L-PLA is used for applications of high mechanical strength and tenacity	L-PLA is more widely used than D-PLA, since L-PLA yields L-lactic acid by hydrolysis, which is the natural lactic acid	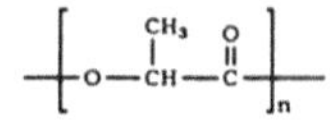
Poly(glycolic acid) (PGA)	Density = 1.50–1.71 g/cm^3 Tensile strength = 60–99 MPa Young's modulus = 6–7 GPa Linear aliphatic Polyiether, Highly crystalline High melting point Low solvent solubility	As suture, it loses mechanical strength after 2–4 weeks after implantation PGA quickly loses crystallinity in admixture with PLA The 50–50 copolymer degrades quicker than PGA or PLA alone	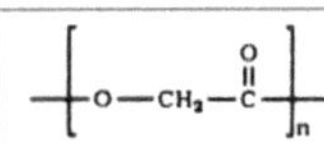
Poly (β-hydroxybutirate)	Density = 1.18–1.23 g/cm^3 Tensile strength = 40 MPa Young's modulus = 3.5–4.0 GPa Xc = 55%		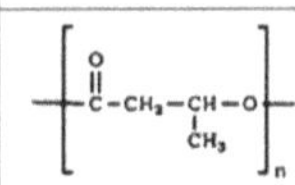
Polivinilpirrolidona (PVP)	Density = 1.2 g/cm^3 Xc = amorphous	Soluble in water and other polar solvents. In powder form it absorbs up to 18% of its mass in the air.	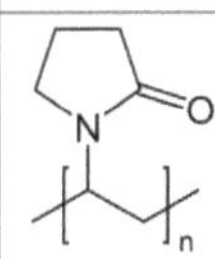
Poly (ε-caprolactone)	Density = 1.11–1.55 g/cm^3 Tensile strength = 20.7–42 MPa Young's modulus = 0.21–0.44 GPa Semicrystalline, High solubility, ε-caprolactone monomer and polycaprolactone are not toxic and are compatible with tissues Low melting point (59–64 °C), Forms polymeric mixtures easily, Excellent processability	Degrades more slowly than PLA, periods higher than 1 year	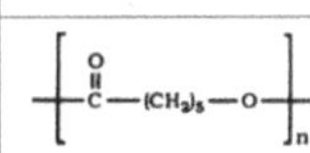

(continued)

Table 5.2 (continued)

Polymer (Initial)	Properties	Limitation	
Poly (hydroxyethyl methacrylate (PHEMA)	Tensile strength = 0.15 MPa Young's modulus = 0.29 GPa Water absorption = 40%		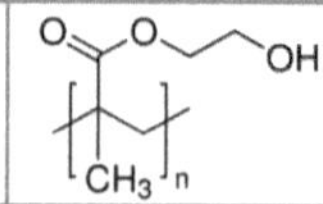
Chitosan	Density = 0.4 g/mL Mn = 69.000 g/mol Tensile strength = 50 MPa Young's modulus 829 ± 357 GPa	Polysaccharide type biopolymer, Molecular structure similar to cellulose, Biocompatibility, Nontoxic, Biodegradable, Antifungal, bacteria, and viruses activity	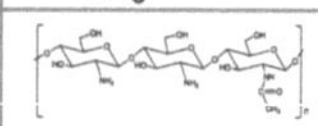

copolymers (made up of two or more kinds of polymers, where at least one of them is hydrophilic), and interpenetrating polymer chain polymer.

Interpenetrating polymers network are hydrogels prepared from the expansion of a gel in a solution containing a second monomer which is then cross-linked within the polymer chain, their chains being then interpenetrated at the molecular level under the action of hydrogen bonds induced by molecular complexes formed by groups which work as hydrogen donors and receptors. As it relates to the gel ionic charges these can be neutral, anionic or cationic, depending on their side groups [28, 29].

5.2.1 *Polymers Used as Hydrogels and Applications of Same as Biomaterials*

Some polymers such as hydrolyzed acrylamide, acrylates (acrylic acid salts), carboxymethylcellulose, alginates are used for forming hydrogels. As polymers are highlighted poly (hydroxyethyl)methacrylate, poly (vinyl alcohol), poly(ethylene glycol), poly(ethylene oxide) and chitosan. As applications, the hydrogels are used the physiological fluids absorption, blood-contacting, timed release drugs, tissue engineering scaffolds, artificial tendon materials, wound healing bioadhesives, artificial kidney membranes, articular cartilage, artificial skin, maxillofacial and sexual organ reconstruction materials. For surgical devices, coating and for producing flexible contact lenses superabsorbent hydrogels shows transparency and visible radiation resistance. [1].

Figure 5.1 illustrates typical polymeric biomaterials applications in the human body.

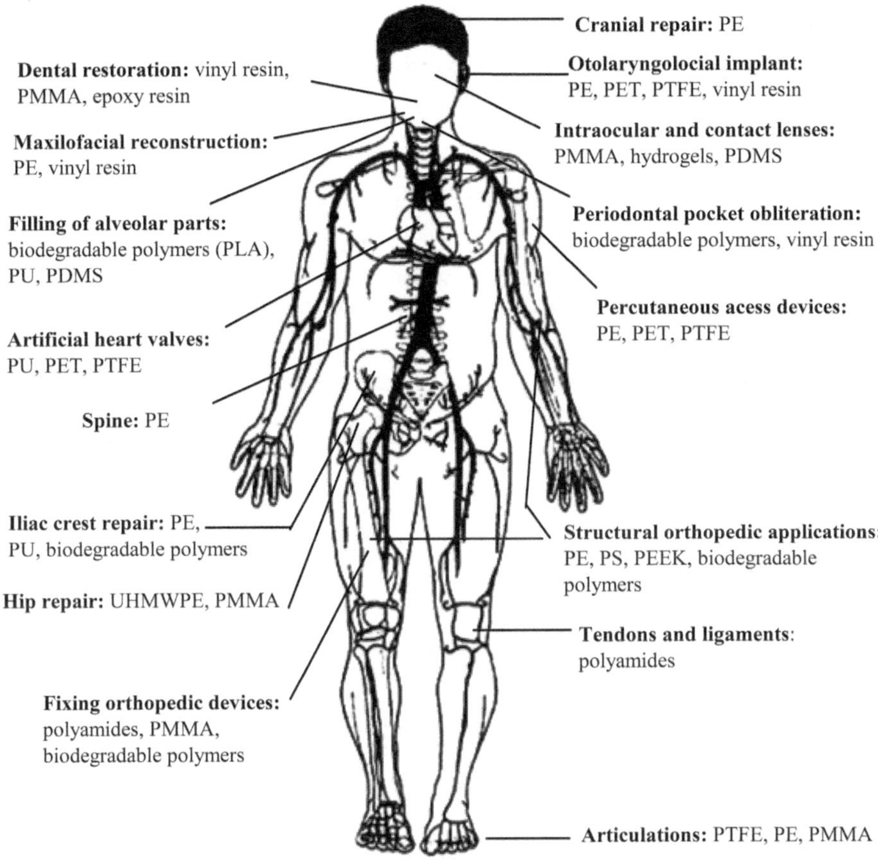

Fig. 5.1 Clinical application of polymeric biomaterials. Adapted [30]

References

1. Ratner, B.D., Hoffman, A.S., Schoen, F.J., Lemons, J.E.: Biomaterials science: an introduction to materials in medicine, 3rd edn. Academic Press, Amsterdam (2013)
2. Park, J.B., Bronzino, J.D.: Biomaterials: principles and applications. CRC Press, Boca Raton (2003)
3. Oréfice, R.L., Pereira, M. de. M., Mansur, H.S.: Biomateriais: fundamentos e aplicações. Cultura Médica, Rio de Janeiro (2006)
4. Akcelrud, L.: Fundamentos da ciência dos polímeros. Manole, São Paulo (2007)
5. Odian, G.: Principles of polymerization, 4th edn. Wiley, New York (2004)
6. Paul, D.R., Newman, S.: Polymer blends. Academic Press, New York (1978)
7. American Society for Testing and Materials. ASTM D 3878—Standard terminology for composite materials. Pennsylvania (2015)
8. Shackelford, J.F.: Introduction to materials science for engineers. Pretice-Hall, New Jersey (2000)

9. Canevarolo, J.R.S.: Ciência dos Polímeros: um texto básico para tecnólogos e engenheiros, 2nd ed. Artliber, São Paulo (2006)
10. Paoli, M.A.de.: Degradação e estabilização de polímeros. Artliber, São Paulo (2008)
11. International Organization For Standardization. ISO 472—Plastics—Vocabulary. Geneva (2013)
12. American Society For Testing Materials. ASTM D6004-04—Standard test method for determining adhesive shear strength of carpet adhesives. Pennsylvania (2011)
13. American Society For Testing Materials. ASTM D883—Terminology relating to plastics. Philadelphia (2012)
14. American Society For Testing Materials. Committee D20 on Plastics, Subcommittee D20.96 on biobased and environmentally degradable plastics. Philadelphia
15. Eglin, D., Alini, M.: Degradable polymeric materials for osteosynthesis: Tutorial. Eur. Cell Mater. **16**, 80–91 (2008)
16. Proikakis, C.S., Mamouzelos, N.J., Tarantili, P.A., Andreopoulos, A.G.: Swelling and hydrolytic degradation of poly(D, L-lactic acid) in aqueous solutions. Polym. Degrad. Stab. **91**(3), 614–619 (2006)
17. Belgacem, M.N., Gandini, A.: Monomers, polymers and composites from renewable resources. Elsevier, Amsterdam (2008)
18. Barbanti, S.H., Zavaglia, C.A.C., Duek, E.A.R.: Polímeros bioreabsorvíveis na engenharia de tecidos. Polímeros. **15**(1), 13–21 (2005)
19. Heller, J.: Drug delivery systems. In: Biomaterials science: an introduction to materials in medicine. Academic Press, 346–356 (1996)
20. Navarro, M., Michiardi, A., Castaño, O., Planell, J.A.: Biomaterials in orthopaedics. J. R. Soc. Interface **5**(27), 1137–1158 (2008)
21. Maia, M., Klein, E.S., Monje, T.V., Pagliosa, C.: Reconstrução da estrutura facial por biomateriais: revisão de literatura. Rev. Bras. Cir. Plást. **25**(3), 566–572 (2010)
22. Sionkowska, A.: Current research on the blends of natural and synthetic polymers as new biomaterials: Review. Prog. Polym. Sci. **36**(9), 1254–1276 (2011)
23. Sell, S.A., Wolfe, P.S., Garg, K., Mccool, J.M., Rodriguez, I.A., Bowlin, G.L.: The use of natural polymers in tissue engineering: A focus on electrospun extracellular matrix analogues. Polymers **2**(4), 522–553 (2010)
24. Mogosanu, G.D., Grumezescu, A.M.: Natural and synthetic polymers for wounds and burns dressing. Int. J. Pharm. **463**, 127–136 (2014)
25. Rinaudo, M.: Main properties and current applications of some polysaccharides as biomaterials. Polym. Int. **57**(3), 397–430 (2008)
26. Kim, Y.D., Kim, S.C.: Effect of chemical structure on the biodegradation of polyurethanes under composting conditions. Polym. Degrad. Stab. **62**(2), 343–352 (1998)
27. Aminabhavi, T.M., Vijaya Kumar Naidu, B., Subha, M.C.S., Sairam, M., Krishna Rao, V.S. K.: Novel chitosan-based pH-sensitive interpenetrating network microgels for the controlled release of cefadroxil. Carbohydr. Polym. **66**, 333–344 (2006)
28. Kopecek, J.: Polymer chemistry: Swell gels. Nature **417**(4), 388–391 (2002)
29. Rosiak, J.M., Janik, I., Kadlubowski, S., Kozicki, M., Kujawa, P., Stasica, P., Ulanski, P.: Radiation formation of hydrogels for biomedical applications. In: Radiation synthesis and modification of polymers for biomedical applications. IAEA, Vienna (2002)
30. Park, J., Lakes, R.S.: Biomaterials: an introduction, 3rd edn. Springer-Verlag, New York (2007)

Chapter 6
Composite Biomaterials

A composite material is defined in accordance with the ASTM D3878-15 Method [1] as a substance consisting of two or more materials, insoluble in one another, which are combined in the intent to obtain a useful engineering material possessing certain properties not shown by the constituents taken separately. Polymeric composites consist of a continuous phase, the polymeric matrix, which is responsible for the composite structure, and a discontinuous phase, dispersed within the matrix, responsible for modifying desired polymer properties or just to reduce costs [2]. The discontinuous phase is usually stiffer and more resistant than the continuous phase.

In order to be considered a composite, a few criteria should be met [3]:

- Constituents are intrinsically insoluble (keeping their identity in the end product), under different forms and/or constitutions and/or properties,
- Properties of interest in the development of a composite need to be notably distinct from those of the constituents,
- Constituents should be present in reasonable amounts (e.g., 5% minimum),
- The different materials (phases) are separated by a microscopic scale interface,
- The obtained (synthetic) composite is generally constituted by admixture and (macroscopic) combination of the constituents.

In composites, the role of the matrix, continuous phase, is to distribute and transfer tensions to fillers (discontinuous phase), besides from protecting it. The matrix nature can be diverse: metallic, polymeric, or ceramic.

As to the dispersed, discontinuous phase, a few structural parameters should be considered when producing a composite since these parameters directly influence the composite properties [2]. These parameters are:

- Kind of constituents,
- Concentration,
- Size and shape,
- Distribution,
- Orientation of constituents.

V. dos Santos et al., *Engineering of Biomaterials*, Topics in Mining, Metallurgy and Materials Engineering, DOI 10.1007/978-3-319-58607-6_6

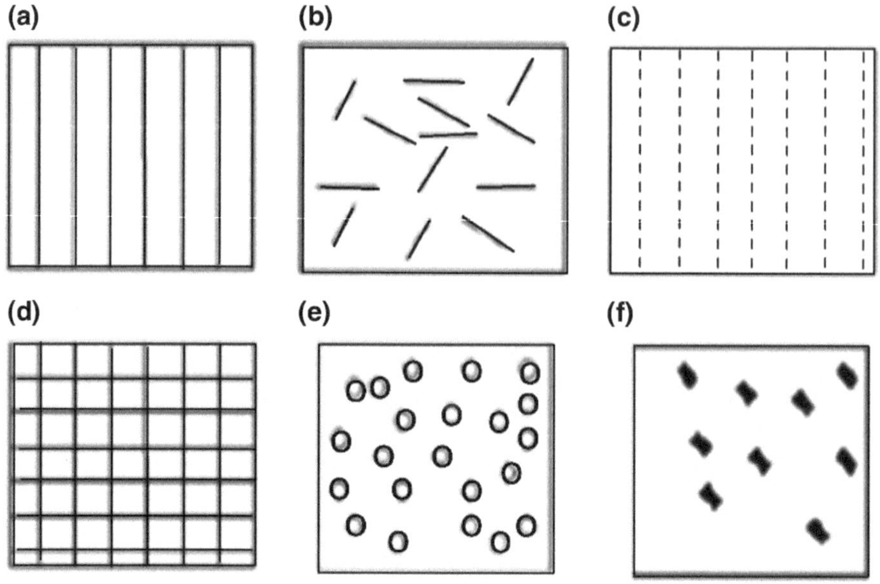

Fig. 6.1 Types of composite materials reinforcement and their orientation in the matrix. **a** Continuous fibers, **b** short and random fibers, **c** oriented short fibers, **d** bidirectional, **e** spherical particles, and **f** flakes [4]

Figures 6.1 and 6.2 display some of the most common disperse phases used as reinforcement for polymeric composites [4, 5].

The above-mentioned structural parameters influence structural performance. The relevance as related to structural performance, economic aspects, and composites' productive cycles in the several fields of interest are displayed in Fig. 6.3 [2].

Between the composite phases there is the interphase and the interface (Fig. 6.4).

The interface represents the space region where the two phases interact by being situated in the interphase. In technical terms, interfacial interactions between matrix and fibers are fundamental for determining overall composite properties. They are responsible for tension transfer from matrices to fibers, besides working crucially as materials corrosion path. The load applied to the matrix has to be transferred to the reinforcement via the interface.

Changes in the matrix/reinforcement interface could influence significantly the properties and performance of composites.

Different thermal and chemical treatments can be applied to improve the interaction/adhesion between matrix/reinforcement. The use of coupling agents, usually chemical compounds, is intended to favor phase interaction. Figure 6.5 illustrates the action of a coupling agent.

The expression adhesion is generally utilized to refer to attraction among substances, and establishes the manifestation of attractive forces among atoms and/or surfaces [2].

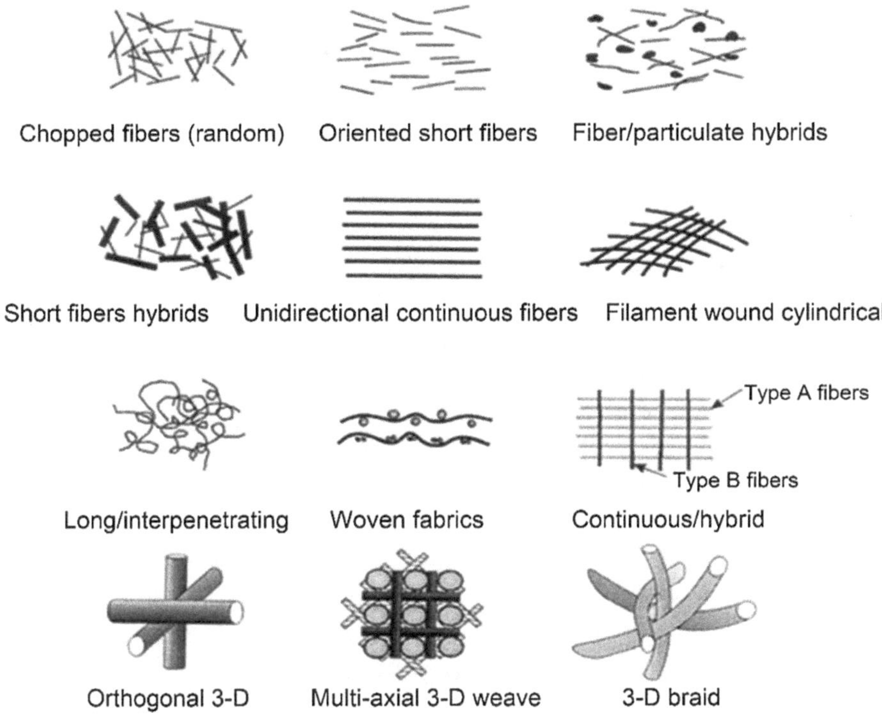

Fig. 6.2 Kinds of reinforcement for composite materials and their orientation in the matrix [5]

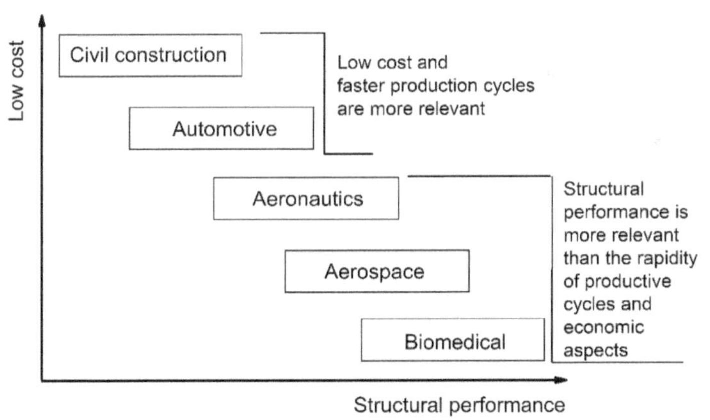

Fig. 6.3 Description of cost and structural performance for composites. Adapted [2]

The nature of adhesion is a function of the presence of fiber superficial functional groups produced by some surface treatment, orientation, atomic arrangement, crystallinity and chemical properties, the matrix chemical constitution, the diffusivity of the elements of each constituent, and the geometrical arrangement of the fibers [2].

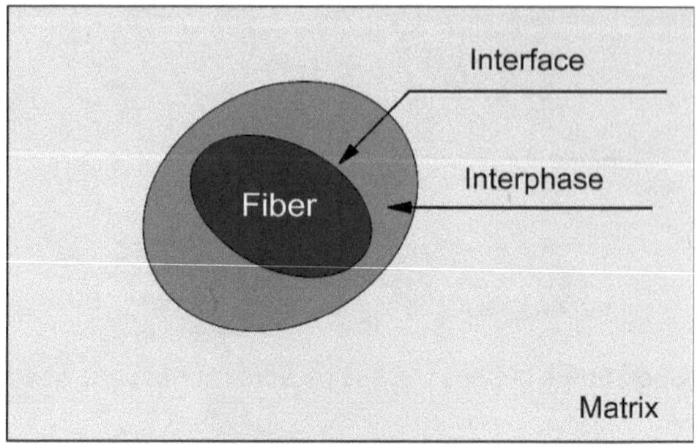

Fig. 6.4 Schematic diagram representing the concepts of interface and interphase for composite materials Adapted [6]

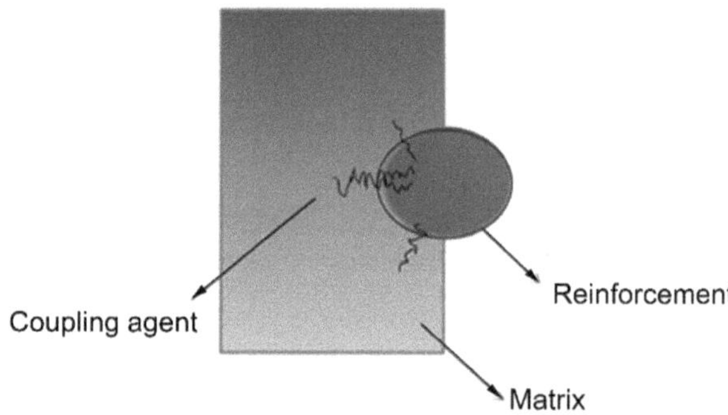

Fig. 6.5 Schematic representation of filler–matrix interaction performed by the coupling agent. Adapted [2]

6.1 Types and Properties of Discontinuous Phases

The main reinforcements utilized in biomaterials are carbon fiber, polymeric fibers, ceramic particles, and glass fibers and particles. Depending on the requirements of the application, the discontinuous phase can be inert or absorbable. According to Ratner [7] numerous studies have been focused on nanocomposites, widening the application of composites for biomaterials and in these, the reinforcement is being based on carbon nanotubes, nanoclays, silica, hydroxyapatite nanoparticles and polyhedral oligomeric silsesquioxane, silicone and oxygen atoms being linked together in cubic form, with silicone atoms occupying the corners (POSS).

Table 6.1 lists the relative figures of some materials' properties in the form of fibers and particles [3].

In some composites the discontinuous phase can be in the form of laminates, consisting of several stacked thin layers ($\sim$1 mm) of fibers impregnated by polymeric resins. A few fiber laminates impregnated by partially cured resin (partially cross linked) are known as pre-preg and can be utilized with other reinforcements of a distinct chemical classification such as metals and ceramics, constituting the so-called hybrid composites. Laminates can exhibit fibers in different orientations and directions.

Table 6.1 Properties of materials in the form of fibers and particles [3]

Material	Tensile modulus (GPa)	Tensile strength (GPa)	Density (g/cm^3)
Steel	200	2.8	7.8
Carbon	585	3.8	1.94
Aramide—kevlar	185	3.4	1.47
UHMWPE	172	3.0	1.0
Nylon	6	1.0	1.14
Polyester	12	1.2	1.39
Hydroxyapatite*	95	0.07	3.16
Bioglass 45S5*	35	0.04	2.66
Glass Fiber (C-S)	72.5	3.45	2.5

*Particle

Fibers woven as tissues of different orientations, angles, and fiber fractions enable to obtain reinforcements that can alter the end properties of composites, so that through the properties isotropy, fiber nature, and characteristics of the polymeric resin it is possible to compare their properties to those of metals (Fig. 6.2).

6.2 Polymeric Phases for Biomaterials

Polymeric matrices most widely used in composites for biomaterials are polysulfone, poly(ether-ether-ketone) (PEEK), ultrahigh molecular weight polyethylene (UHMWPE), polytetrafluoroethylene (PTFE), poly(methylmethacrylate) (PMMA), and epoxy resins. Among the bioresorbable polymers in composites poly (lactic acid) is highlighted.

The properties of polymeric matrices for composites are described below.

Polysulfone and poly(ether-ether-ketone) (PEEK)—high thermal, mechanical, and chemical resistance. Resistance to hydrolysis and to super heated steam. Good wear resistance, easy machinability, and high resistance to intensive energy radiations. The ASTM F2026 Method standardizes the specifications of PEEK for application in surgical implants [8].

Ultrahigh molecular weight polyethylene (UHMWPE)—this is a member of the polyethylene family of polymers with the repeat unit $[C_2H_4]_n$, with n denoting the degree of polymerization. The UHMWPEs used in orthopedic applications typically have a molecular weight between 2 and 6 million with a degree of polymerization between 71,000 and 214,000 [9, 10]. UHMWPE is a linear (non-branched) semi-crystalline polymer which can be described as a two-phase composite of crystalline and amorphous phases. The crystalline phase contains chains folded into highly oriented lamellae, with the crystals being orthorhombic in structure [11].

Epoxy resins—high adhesion to fibers, solvent resistance, low contraction, low fracture toughness, high flow, and temperature resistance.

6.3 Metallic Phases for Biomaterials

Silver-containing composites are objects of study due to the antimicrobial effect of silver against a huge variety of bacteria, fungi, protozoa, and viruses [12]. This metal is mainly used as micro and nanoparticles incorporated into polymeric materials in the medical field for treatments of burn, infections, and skin injuries. In devices like catheters, silver can prevent bacterial colonization during use [13, 14]. Stevens et al reported on the antimicrobial effect of catheter coatings containing silver nanoparticles and blood clotting on contact [13]. Antimicrobial coatings are especially important in connection with indwelling catheters with a high risk of bacterial line infections, such as central venous catheters (CVCs). This study performed in vitro with fresh platelet-rich blood plasma (PRP) from 5 different healthy volunteer donors, clearly pointed out that: (i) the presence of silver nanoparticles correlates with accelerated thrombin formation upon contact of the coating with PRP, (ii) platelet activation is stronger as a result from the contact with silver nanoparticle-containing coatings as compared to other coatings which are devoid of silver. A series of titration experiments, in which the potential effect of silver ions is mimicked, revealed that the observed activation of blood platelets can be best explained through a collision mechanism. The results suggest that platelets that collide with silver, exposed at the surface, become activated without adhering to the surface [13, 14].

All and every development employing metals that could compromise human and animal health and environmental preservation should have its results determined and checked by competent agencies of teaching institutions, in the case of universities (Biosafety and Ethics Committee) or health surveillance.

Biosafety is a body of actions turned to the prevention, reduction, or elimination of risks inherent to the activities of research, production, teaching, development, technology, and service rendering directed to human and animal health, to environmental preservation, and to the quality of results [15].

6.4 Ceramic Phases for Biomaterials

In polymeric biomaterials for bone implant the addition of bioglass, hydroxyapatite, and other calcium phosphates particles aims at enhancing the matrix biocompatibility and elastic modulus. In this way, the composite mechanical properties are rendered similar to those of bone, contributing to the reduction of the stress-shielding phenomenon [16].

The combination of calcium phosphates with proteins such as gelatin and collagen results in compounds with physical, mechanical, and biological characteristics similar to those of human bones [16].

Table 6.2 Main composite constituents for use in the biomedical field [17]

Particles	Fiber	Matrix
Inorganic Glass Alumina	*Polymers* Aromatic Polyamides (aramids) UHMWPE Polyesters Polyolefins PTFE	*Thermosets* Epoxy Polyacrylates Polymethacrylates Polyesters Silicones
Organic Polyacrylate Polymethacrylate	*Resorbable polymers* Polylactide, and its copolymers with polyglycolide Silk Collagen *Inorganic* Carbon Glass Hydroxyapatite Tricalcium phosphate	*Thermoplastics* Polyolefins (PP, PE) UHMWPE Polysulfones Poly(ether ketones) Polyesters *Inorganic* Hydroxyapatite Glass ceramics Calciumcarbonateceramics Calciumphosphateceramics Carbono Steel Titanium *Resorbable polymers* Polylactide, polyglycolide and their copolymers Polydioxanone

6.5 Selection of Properties Between Materials and Tissues

When selecting a composite biomaterial it is important to consider the property differences between the biomaterial and the tissues. Significant differences in specific properties, such as tensile strength could lead to unsuccessful implant or prosthesis (stress shield).

Table 6.2 lists the main composite constituents for use in the biomedical field [17].

Figure 6.6 illustrates the properties of Young's modulus and mechanical resistance of materials, composites and tissues while Fig. 6.7 shows the properties of some composites with polymers, metals, and ceramics.

Figure 6.8 illustrates typical composites biomaterials applications in the human body.

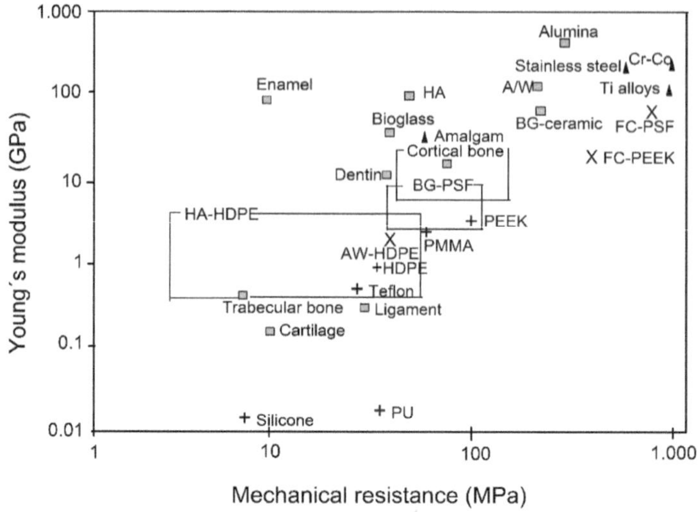

Fig. 6.6 Mechanical properties of some biomaterials: (*Plus*) Polymers, (*Green-filled box*) Living tissues, (*Grey-filled box*) Ceramic, (*Traingle*) Metals and (X) Composites [18]

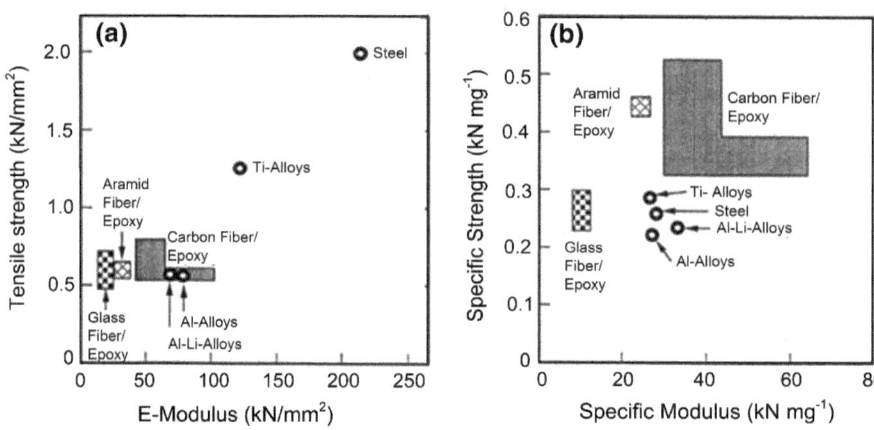

Fig. 6.7 Properties of **a** tensile strength x E-modulus and **b** specific strength x specific modulus of some composites, materials [19]

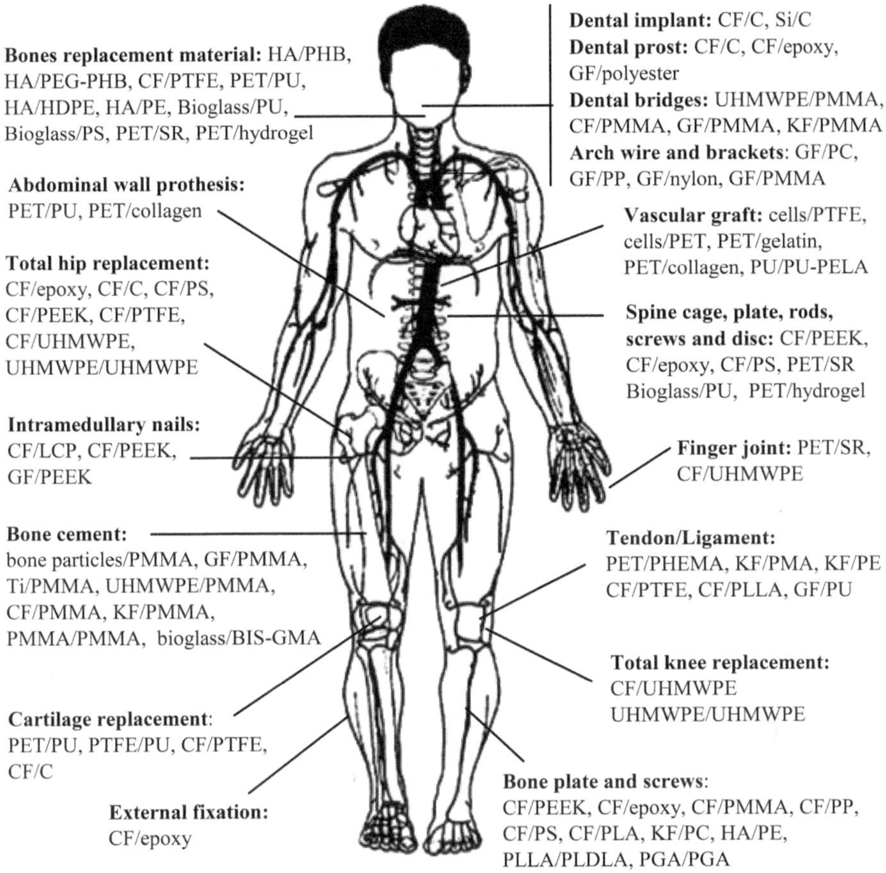

Fig. 6.8 Clinical applications of composites biomaterials [20]

References

1. American Society For Testing And Materials. ASTM D 3878—Standard Terminology for Composite Materials. EUA (2015)
2. Neto, F.L., Pardini, L.C.: Compósitos Estruturais: Ciência e Tecnologia. Edgard Blücher, São Paulo (2006)
3. Peters, S.T.: Handbook of composites, 2nd edn. Chapman & Hall, London (1998)
4. Ventura, A.M.F.M.: Os compósitos e sua aplicação na Reabilitação de Estruturas metálicas. C. Tecn. Mat. **21**(3–4), 10–19 (2009)
5. Gupta, M.C., Gupta, A.P.: Polymer composite. New Age International, New Delhi (2007)
6. Burakowski, L., Rezende, M.: Modificação da rugosidade de fibras de carbono por método químico para aplicação em compósitos poliméricos. Polímeros **11**(2), 51–57 (2001)
7. Ratner, B.D., Hoffman, A.S., Schoen, F.J., Lemons, J.E.: Biomaterials science: an introduction to materials in medicine, 3rd edn. Academic Press, Amsterdam (2013)
8. American Society For Testing And Materials. ASTM F2026—Standard Specification for Poly ether ether ketone (PEEK) Polymers for Surgical Implant Applications. EUA (2014)

9. Li, S., Burstein, A.H.: Current concepts review: Ultra high molecular weight polyethylene. J. Bone Joint Surg. Am. **76A**, 1080–1090 (1994)
10. Kurtz, S.: The UHMWPE handbook: ultra-high molecular weight polyethylene in total joint replacement. Academic Press, New York (2004)
11. Lin, L., Argon, A.S.: Structure and plastic deformation of polyethylene. J. Mater. Sci. **29**, 294–323 (1994)
12. Nordberg, G.F., Fowler, B.A., Anordberg, M.: Handbook on the toxicology of metals: general consideratiron, 4th edn. Academic Press, San Diego (2014)
13. Stevens, K.N., Crespo-Biel, O., Van Den Bosch, E.E., Dias, A.A., Knetsch, M.L., Aldenhoff, Y.B., Van Der Veen, F.H., Maessen, J.G., Stobberingh, E.E., Koole, L.H.: The relationship between the antimicrobial effect of catheter coatings containing silver nanoparticles and the coagulation of contacting blood. Biomaterials **30**, 3682–3690 (2009)
14. Stevens, K.N.J., Croes, S., Boersma, S., Stobberingh, E.E., Van Der Marel, C., Van Der Veen, F.H., Knetsch, M.L.W., Koole, L.H.: Hydrophilic surface coatings with embedded biocidal silver nanoparticles and sodium heparin for central venous catheters. Biomaterials **32**, 1264–1269 (2011)
15. Teixeira, P., Valle, S.: Biossegurança: uma abordagem multidisciplinar, 2nd edn. Fiocruz, Rio de Janeiro (2010)
16. Habraken, W.J.E., Wolke, J.G.C., Jansen, J.A.: Ceramic composites as matrices and scaffolds for drug delivery in tissue engineering. Adv. Drug Deliv. Rev. **59**, 234–248 (2007)
17. Patel, N.R., Gohil, P.P.: A review on biomaterials: Scope, applications & human anatomy significance. IJETAE **2**(4), 91–101 (2012)
18. Oréfice, R.L., Pereira, M. de. M., Mansur, H.S.: Biomaterials: fundamentos e aplicações. Cultura Médica, Rio de Janeiro (2006)
19. Polymer Science Learning Center. Introduction to fiber production and their incorporation into composites. Available at: http://www.pslc.ws/macrog/mpm/composit/fiber/. Accessed Jan 2017
20. Park, J., Lakes, R.S.: Biomaterials: an introduction, 3rd edn. Springer, New York (2007)

Chapter 7
Biomaterials Sterilization Methods

Following the choice of the ideal biomaterial for a certain application, it is necessary to sterilize it. Sterilization is the final step in the manufacture of any biomaterial, being responsible for microorganism removal from the material surface. Since it is an important process related to the future application and the consequences for the human body, the effect of sterilization and the possible modifications at the material's surface and characteristics should be clearly understood and assessed.

Metallic biomaterials, owing to their characteristics and high temperature resistance can be sterilized by practically all of the sterilization processes. However, depending on the material composition, autoclave, for example, could cause corrosion on some biomaterials, chiefly those of high carbon concentration [1].

Ceramic biomaterials, as well as metallic ones, are also resistant to most of the conventional sterilization methods. However, steam sterilization applied to bioceramics, as is the case with zirconia, could foster phase transformation in its crystalline structure [1].

Most of the polymeric biomaterials exhibit relatively low melting temperatures and are susceptible to degradation and/or morphological modifications at high temperatures. This fact hinders the utilization of high temperatures requiring sterilization methods. Owing to these facts, the polymeric biomaterials class requires higher care in the choice of the best sterilization method in order to keep intact all of the biomaterial properties after the process [2].

The use of heat as steam and radiation are well known for affecting mechanical and optical polymer properties. Sterilization by chemical agents can affect medical grade polymers rendering them toxic materials besides providing insufficient sterility. Ethylene oxide is compatible with numerous materials (polymers, metals, ceramics, and composites), however, toxic residues could remain in the material after sterilization, hindering removal. Owing to the free radicals generated during the process hydrogen peroxide plasma can react with the polymer chain and onset the degradation process [3, 4].

V. dos Santos et al., *Engineering of Biomaterials*, Topics in Mining, Metallurgy and Materials Engineering, DOI 10.1007/978-3-319-58607-6_7

The choice of the sterilization method is of paramount importance for the biomaterial success under various aspects to be considered, among which are the integrity of the biomaterial properties and of the surface characteristics that are directly related to the performance of the material and the biocompatibility.

7.1 Sterilization Methods

Sterilization methods applied to biomaterials can be grouped into physical and chemical methods. Physical sterilization methods are characterized by the use of various forms of heat and a few kinds of radiation. Chemical methods are associated with chemical compounds interaction. To each of these methods are attributed particular characteristics and specific applications to eliminate body harmful microbial life [5].

Before starting the sterilization process, no matter the chosen method, it is necessary and of paramount importance that the biomaterial undergoes a cleaning process. Cleaning is responsible for the removal of materials resulting from processing or handling, for example, dust and organic matter. This process can be performed manually or by ultrasonic devices, both with the aid of specific detergents and distilled or deionized water, followed by drying [1, 6].

Figure 7.1 illustrates the process steps to which biomaterials should be submitted before being utilized as biomaterial.

It is important to point out that the expression disinfection cannot be confounded with sterilization. Disinfection reduces microbial load, but does not eliminate it completely, therefore does not promote the required safety level for biomaterials application. Ethanol, for example, is largely employed for disinfection since it

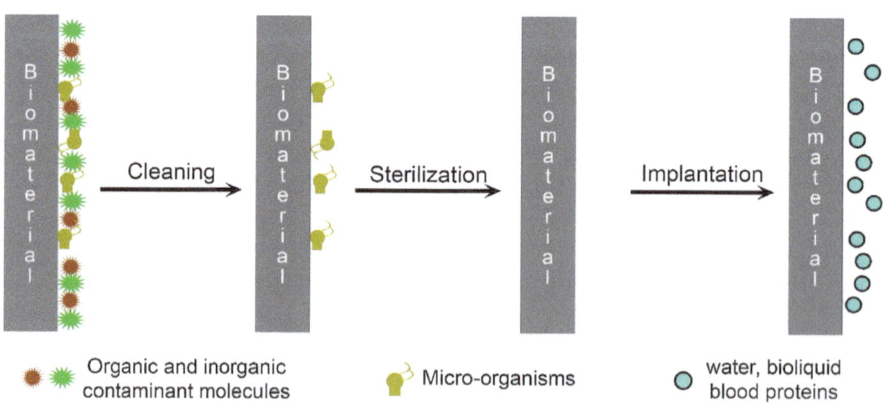

Fig. 7.1 Illustration of a biomaterial surface during the cleaning, sterilization and implantation process

possesses a protein dehydration and coagulation action and does not work on endospores of most of bacteria species; therefore it cannot be utilized as a sterilization method, just as a disinfection tool [7, 8].

7.1.1 Ethylene Oxide

Sterilization by ethylene oxide is one of the most widely used methods for biomaterials' sterilization due to the high process efficacy at low temperatures and high penetration power. The process occurs in the interior of a chamber with a combination of relative humidity varying from 40 to 80%, ethylene oxide gas concentration of 450–1200 mg L^{-1}, temperature in the range of 40–65 °C and exposure time varying from a few hours up to a few days [9, 10]. The sterilization process should assure that all parameters are provided in the interior of the chamber to secure the required sterility to the biomaterial while not causing any harmful effect on its properties and functionality.

Process parameters with ethylene oxide that should be carefully evaluated for biomaterials sterilization are those which can affect the product and the package where the material is conditioned and those related to transfer rate. Vacuum levels, vacuum cycles levels, chamber temperature, gas concentration, exposure time to humidity, and any diluents can affect the biomaterial structure and alter its characteristics [5].

Residual ethylene oxide after the sterilization process is toxic and therefore it is mandatory to perform degasification steps in order to eliminate all gas residues which could remain on the biomaterial. Complete removal of gas residual remains could prove difficult, especially for porous materials. Besides, ethylene oxide gas is chemically reactive and leads to changes in polymers structure.

Remaining residues on the material after ethylene oxide sterilization process should comply with the limits imposed by regulating agencies, such as Food and Drug Administration (FDA). Residua maximum limit for ethylene oxide-sterilized materials and their by-products is listed in Table 7.1 [11].

Monitoring ethylene oxide remaining after sterilization was checked for poly (ether-ether-ketone) samples by means of the thermogravimetry technique at different heating rates in a paper by Savaris and co-workers (2016) (Chemical and Thermal Evaluation of Commercial and Medical Grade PEEK Sterilization by Ethylene Oxide) [12]. The studied sterilization process consisted in samples sterilized with different parameters, among which, samples undergoing sterilization only, sterilized, aerated and hyperventilated samples and sterilized, aerated and hyperventilated and aerated again for 24 h samples. These changes in parameters were scrutinized in the light of the fact that aeration and hyperventilation processes are responsible for reduction or removal of ethylene oxide from the samples.

Results of the remaining ethylene oxide test showed that for all samples experimental values were higher than the maximum FDA allowed limit. And

Table 7.1 Maximum residue limits for ethylene oxide, ethylene chlorohydrin and ethylene glycol (parts per million) [11]

Device type	Ethylene oxide	Ethylene chlorohydrin	Ethylene glycol
Implant:			
Small (<10 g)	250	250	5000
Medium (10–100 g)	100	100	2000
Large (>100 g)	25	25	500
Intrauterine devices	5	10	10
Intraocular lenses	25	25	500
Devices contacting:			
Mucosa	250	250	5000
Blood (ex vivo)	25	25	250
Skin	250	250	5000
Surgical scrub sponges	25	250	500

among the tested heating rates in Thermogravimetric analysis (5, 10, 20 °C min^{-1}), the best result was obtained for 10 °C min^{-1}.

Knowing sterilization process parameters and understanding how they interact with materials are key requisites when it comes to choose the best method not to modify biomaterials properties.

The combination of temperature and humidity utilized in the sterilization process can hinder the bioabsorbable polymers sterilization with possible degradation and structural modification. Other polymers which are affected by the ethylene oxide process include some polyacrilates, such as polymethylmetacrylate and a few styrene resins, such as for example polystyrene and styrene acrylonitrile [5].

In a study with electrospun PLLA fibers, the ethylene oxide sterilization modified morphology, however no alteration occurred in number average molecular weight (Mn) and weight average molecular weight (Mw). Sterilized PCL nanofibers had reduced contact angle and rendered the sample translucid and brittle, making it impossible to perform mechanical tests [10].

7.1.2 Hydrogen Peroxide Plasma

Hydrogen peroxide plasma sterilization is a promising sterilization method and a relatively new technology, marketed under the brand name STERRAD® by Advanced Sterilization Products (ASP), a business affiliated of Johnson & Johnson. The process is quick, efficient and performed in a low humidity and temperature environment.

The sterilization cycle by hydrogen peroxide plasma encompasses five main steps: vacuum, injection, diffusion, plasma, and ventilation. In short, vacuum is applied for removing air from the chamber interior, injection and hydrogen peroxide concentration in liquid form in the condensation and vaporization unit, gas diffusion in the chamber interior, plasma formation by radiofrequency and lastly, ventilation and decomposition of remaining free radicals into water and oxygen [1, 5].

The advantages of the hydrogen peroxide plasma sterilization process are related to the short sterilization circuit, low temperature and humidity, free from toxic chemical residues, irrelevant environmental impact and wide compatibility with several materials [13].

Sterilization can be applied to metals, elastomers, silicone, and a wide variety of polymers. However, liquids, oils, powders, cellulose, cotton, and other H_2O_2—absorbing materials are not recommended for this technique, as well as most biological tissues [1].

A further important aspect which should be observed in plasma sterilization is that this process can cause modifications on the biomaterial surface since hydrogen peroxide is a strong oxidant and the gas plasma has the ability to alter solid surfaces by etching and deposition which depend on the adopted process parameters. For polymers, surface modifications, such as increase in wettability and adhesion properties can occur after sterilization by hydrogen peroxide plasma [1].

A comparative study of the hydrogen peroxide plasma and ethylene oxide sterilization methods was performed on orthopedic PLLA implants. Results demonstrated that hydrogen peroxide plasma sterilization did not alter the molar mass and both methods led to physical aging signs as evidenced by thermal and mechanical analyses. For both methods no significant morphological and chemical alterations were observed. However, hydrogen peroxide traces were observed on the PLLA sample [14].

7.1.3 Autoclave

Autoclave sterilization is an old sterilization method, driven by the variables temperature, pressure, and exposure time. Process steps include: preparation, loading, air removal, heating, sterilization, exhaust, and drying. The process exposes living organisms to minimum temperature conditions of 121 °C, pressure of 1.2 atm and exposure periods of 15–20 min, depending on the size and mass of the devices to be sterilized [15, 16].

Saturated steam is efficient above the temperature of 105 °C and the humidity and heat generated in the interior of the autoclave should penetrate the whole of the biomaterial in order to secure sterility [1].

In spite of the autoclave sterilization method being quick and free from toxic products when compared with other methods such as is the case with ethylene oxide, one of the disadvantages of the process is related to the application for biomaterials having high temperatures sensitivity properties [15].

The autoclave method can be applied to sterilize most of metals and ceramics and a few heat resistant polymers, such as is the case with acetal, nylons, polycarbonate, polypropylene, polysulfones, and polytetrafluoroethylene [1].

In some cases, autoclave sterilization can modify materials properties, such as for example, cause corrosion on metals, phase changes in ceramics, and degradation in polymers.

According to studies performed on hydroxyapatite particles, the autoclave sterilization process did not promote alterations in the material morphology when it is submitted to autoclave procedures. In the same study, it was also reported that this sterilization method when applied to titanium dioxide nanotubes affected osteoblasts adhesion, proliferation, and activity [16].

POSS polyurethane nanocomposites biomaterials: a no degradable POSS-PCU with an aromatic hard segment and carbonate-based soft segment, and a biodegradable POSS-PCL based on an aliphatic hard segment and caprolactone soft segment were autoclave-sterilized. The POSS-PCU sample did not undergo alterations by the sterilization process however the POSS-PCL sample lost all structural integrity due to severe process conditions and probably to the polymer biodegradable nature [17].

7.1.4 Irradiation Sterilization

In the irradiation sterilization method, the material is packaged and exposed to a radiation dose emitted by electrons or photons penetrating the package and inactivating the microbial load present in the material so as to promote sterilization. For the sterilization to be efficient the main process parameters to be evaluated are the sterilization dose and the number of cycles by process.

According to the international standard for radiation sterilization (ANSI/AAMI/ISO 11137-2:2013) [18], radiation sterilization modes include gamma rays, electron beam and X-rays, the gamma rays and electron beam sterilization being the most widely used methods for biomaterials.

Gamma radiation sterilization utilizes cobalt-60 (^{60}Co) or cesium-137 (^{137}Cs) as radiation sources. ^{60}Co delivers gamma rays with energy of 1173 and 1332 MeV and has useful life of 5.27 years, while the energy generated by ^{137}Cs is 0.662 MeV and its half-life is 30.1 years [1].

The usually employed dose for gamma sterilization is 25 kGy and the maximum temperature varies from 30 to 40 °C. During the sterilization process, the radiation is able to penetrate packages and the biomaterial, gamma ray penetration being inversely proportional to the density of the material [10].

Electron beam radiation is obtained by electrons accelerators, generally of the kind of DC accelerators and radiofrequency-based accelerators. For the DC accelerators, the best known commercial devices are distributed by Dynamitron R and the Insulated Core Transformer, which can supply up to 5 MeV. For higher energies radiofrequency accelerators, able to attain 10 MeV, are used [1].

Energy generated by electrons accelerators required for sterilization varies from 5 to 10 MeV and the dose is in the range of 10–50 kGy (for biomaterials the recommended dose is 25 kGy) and the power of penetration is lower than that by gamma ray sterilization [10].

The short sterilization time and the low temperature used in radiation processes favor the application for numerous heat sensitive materials. However, when applied to polymeric biomaterials, these can cause chemical modifications resulting from free radical interactions with the polymeric chain leading to cross-linking or chain scission, besides physical modifications such as molecular weight, embrittlement, decoloration, and fusion [19].

A study directed to the evaluation of the effect of gamma radiation and electron beam (5–200 kGy) sterilization on poly(ether-block-amide) (PEBA) biomaterials was performed aiming at assessing the influence of the processes on the mechanical, structural, chemical, and thermal properties. The different doses evaluated in the radiation sterilization processes led to undeniable changes in the biomaterial characteristics. In the mechanical tests, tensile strength and percentage elongation at break exhibited a slight increase for low radiation doses and drastic reduction consequent to high radiation dose. Stiffness increased with the increase in radiation dose and melt flow index level had increased melting resistance, pointing to increased molar mass. Upon thermal analysis by the technique of differential exploratory calorimetry no changes in thermal transitions could be observed [20].

Increased cross-link density was observed as a result of increased dose electron beam radiation, as well as trans-vinylene unsaturations and carbonyl group concentration was observed by FTIR for both processes. The surface became rougher with increased radiation dose as well as color turned more yellowish. In short, gamma ray sterilization caused more adverse effects on PEBA properties as compared with electron beam radiation [20].

Case study—Metallic biomaterial sterilization
Influence of various sterilization procedures on TiO_2 nanotubes used for biomedical devices [21]

In the class of metallic biomaterials, titanium is thoroughly highlighted as a biomaterial owing to its good mechanical properties and anticorrosive and biocompatible surface properties due to the formation of a titanium dioxide protective layer. One of the applications of titanium as biomaterial is directed to the replacement of hard tissues and to provide for these applications, titanium should have its chemical, physical, morphological, and mechanical properties well defined in order to promote the best osseointegration, cell growth, and biofunctionality results.

Surface properties of titanium dioxide nanotubes (TiO_2 NT) were evaluated after autoclave, hydrogen peroxide plasma, and ultraviolet radiation sterilization in seeking for the best sterilization method for this material.

Surface wettability was assessed by contact angle measurement on flat and nanotubular titanium samples. The initial figure for flat samples contact angle was 77° and after sterilization this figure decreased to 55° in autoclaved samples, 34° for ultraviolet-sterilized samples while plasma samples were practically

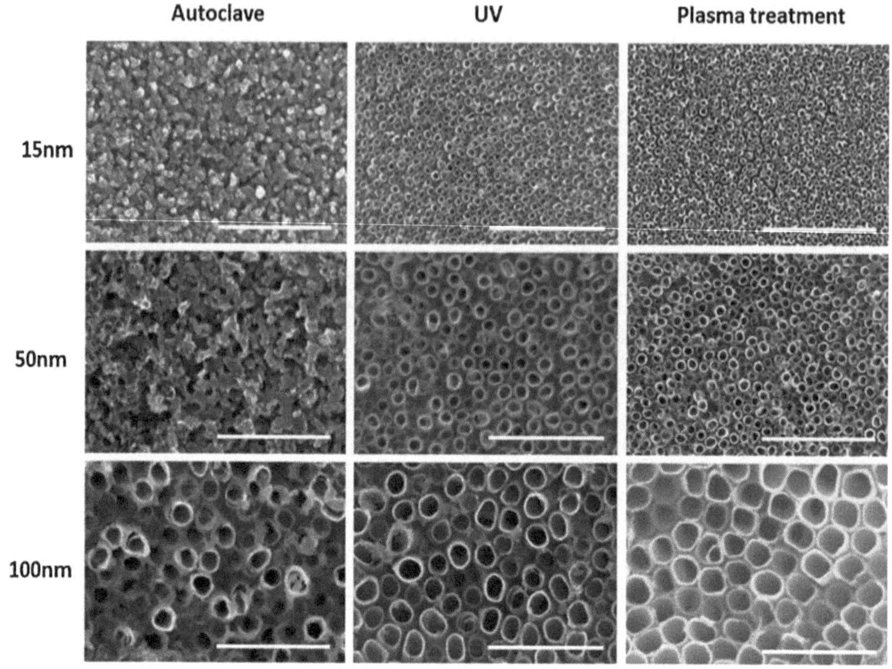

Fig. 7.2 SEM images of nanotubes with 15, 50 and 100 nm in diameter after sterilization. Scale bar: 1 μm [21]

superhydrophilic. For nanotubular samples, all sterilization processes rendered the samples surface hydrophilic.

SEM analyses were also performed in order to assess the surface characteristics of nanotubular titanium samples (15, 50 and 100 nm) (Fig. 7.2). Autoclave sterilization significantly impaired the samples' surface characteristics, the 100 nm titanium being the less damaged sample by the sterilization process, however with some evidence of structure sinterization and increased thickness of the nanotubes walls. The lower diameter samples were the most thoroughly damaged, the titanium 50 nm nanotubes were destroyed and exhibited low porosity. On its turn, the structure of the 15 nm sample was sinterized and the tubes collapsed, totally losing tubular characteristic. Following UV sterilization nanotubes' order was disrupted while after plasma sterilization no modification could be observed.

AFM analysis also indicated surface modifications for autoclave-sterilized samples, with disruption and evidence of nanotubes broken and closed at the top. The remaining sterilization processes did not show influence on the surface morphology by AFM. Roughness was tested on titanium flat samples which exhibited at first 11.8 $\pm$ 3 nm, the results showing increase after autoclave (23 $\pm$ 2 nm), ultraviolet (37.3 $\pm$ 3 nm), and plasma (35.7 $\pm$ 2 nm) sterilization. Similar values were obtained for the roughness of 100 nm diameter titanium nanotubes.

It is well known that autoclave is a rigid process for numerous biomaterials. however the vast majority of metals can be sterilized by this technique owing to their characteristics and resistance at high temperatures.

However, modifications observed on TiO_2 NT after the autoclave sterilization process could be related to the combined effect of heat and humidity that leads to the titanium nanotubes crystallization. Water vapor molecules could have promoted some interaction with the amorphous titanium nanotubes walls, which led to condensation, this also possibly working as a catalyst to foster the TiO_6^{-2} octahedral rearrangement. Finally, it could be ascertained that autoclave sterilization is not suitable for sterilizing TiO_2 NT.

Case study—Ceramic biomaterial sterilization
Optimal sterilization method for the zirconia/alumina composites used for total hip replacements [22]

Ceramic biomaterials such as for example zirconia and alumina which together can build a composite for application in hip prostheses can be sterilized by saturated steam, dry heat, and ethylene oxide and gamma radiation. However, steam and dry heat sterilization methods can possibly cause phase changes and roughness at the surface due to the yttria-stabilized zirconia besides increasing wear, leading to biomaterial failure. Owing to these possible changes, sterilization methods by ethylene oxide and gamma radiation are usually employed for sterilizing zirconia-, alumina- or ceramic components-containing biomaterials [22].

Zirconia/alumina hip heads were sterilized by ethylene oxide and gamma radiation at doses of 25 and 50 kGy. Results revealed that 50 kGy gamma sterilization promoted sterilization at the surface and in the interior of samples, while the 25 kGy dose and the ethylene oxide sterilization sterilized just the surface. There were no zirconia phase changes from tetragonal to monocyclic which could be envisaged by X-rays diffraction after the different sterilization methods, as well as no mechanical alterations could be observed by means of biaxial flexure strength measurements.

Case study—Polymeric biomaterial sterilization
Influence of different sterilization processes on the properties of commercial poly(lactic acid) [23]

The care in sterilizing polymer biomaterials is related to the thermal and chemical characteristics of these materials which are sensible to high temperatures and humidity.

Poly(lactic acid) (PLA) is one of the most sought-after polymers for application in the biomaterials field owing to its characteristics of good mechanical properties, ease of processing in conventional equipment, high transparency and biocompatibility.

PLA films properties were assessed before different sterilization processes (ethylene oxide, hydrogen peroxide plasma, autoclave, gamma rays radiation, and electron beam radiation) (Table 7.2), aiming at evaluating the effect caused by these processes on the PLA morphological, physical, chemical, and thermal properties.

Table 7.2 Hygienization and sterilization parameters applied to PLA [23]

Sample	Process	Parameters
PLA_C	Control	No process
PLA_H	Hygienization	Enzymatic detergent and water (2 mL/L), temperature of cleaning 50 °C, temperature of rinsing 45 °C, process time 45 min
PLA_{SETO}	Sterilization by ethylene oxide	Temperature 55 °C, time 6 h 30 min
PLA_{SSS}	Sterilization by saturated steam—autoclaving	Temperature 121 °C, pressure 2 bar, time 20 min
PLA_{SH2O2}	Sterilization by hydrogen peroxide plasma	Temperature 45–55 °C, time 28 min
PLA_{SEB}	Sterilization by electron beam radiation	Dose 25 kGy
PLA_{SGR}	Sterilization by gamma radiation	Dose 25 kGy

Optical microscopy data after the different sterilization processes indicated that saturated steam sterilization led to modification on PLAsss surface, with thorn out regions and appearance of holes (Fig. 7.3). These surface modifications could be related to process conditions (T, P) which are prone to trigger polymer degradation. The other sterilization processes did not cause surface modifications.

Besides surface modifications, chemical structure modifications were observed in the PLAsss sample by the Fourier transform infrared spectroscopy (FTIR) technique. The appearance of an absorption band in the 3500–3000 cm^{-1} region, related to the −OH group stretching points out to the onset of the hydrolytic degradation process. Further sterilization processes did not cause modifications related to PLA degradation.

A further hint which corroborates PLA degradation is the sample color change. Colorimetric analysis, together with FTIR analysis and films images, corroborate PLA degradation with color change from transparent to white (Fig. 7.4).

By thermal analysis it was possible to observe variations in glass transition temperature (Tg), cold crystallization temperature (Tcc), melting temperature (Tm) and index of crystallinity for all the sterilization processes, the saturated steam sterilization being the process leading to the deepest modifications. Tg and Tcc values were not observed for the saturated steam sterilized sample due to a possible crystallization, since the PLA crystallization temperature is around 106 °C and this temperature was exceeded during the sterilization process.

Finally, by studying the different sterilization processes assayed on PLA and in view of the possible modifications caused by these processes on the biomaterial characteristics, only saturated steam sterilization caused damages which precluded its utilization for sterilizing this kind of material.

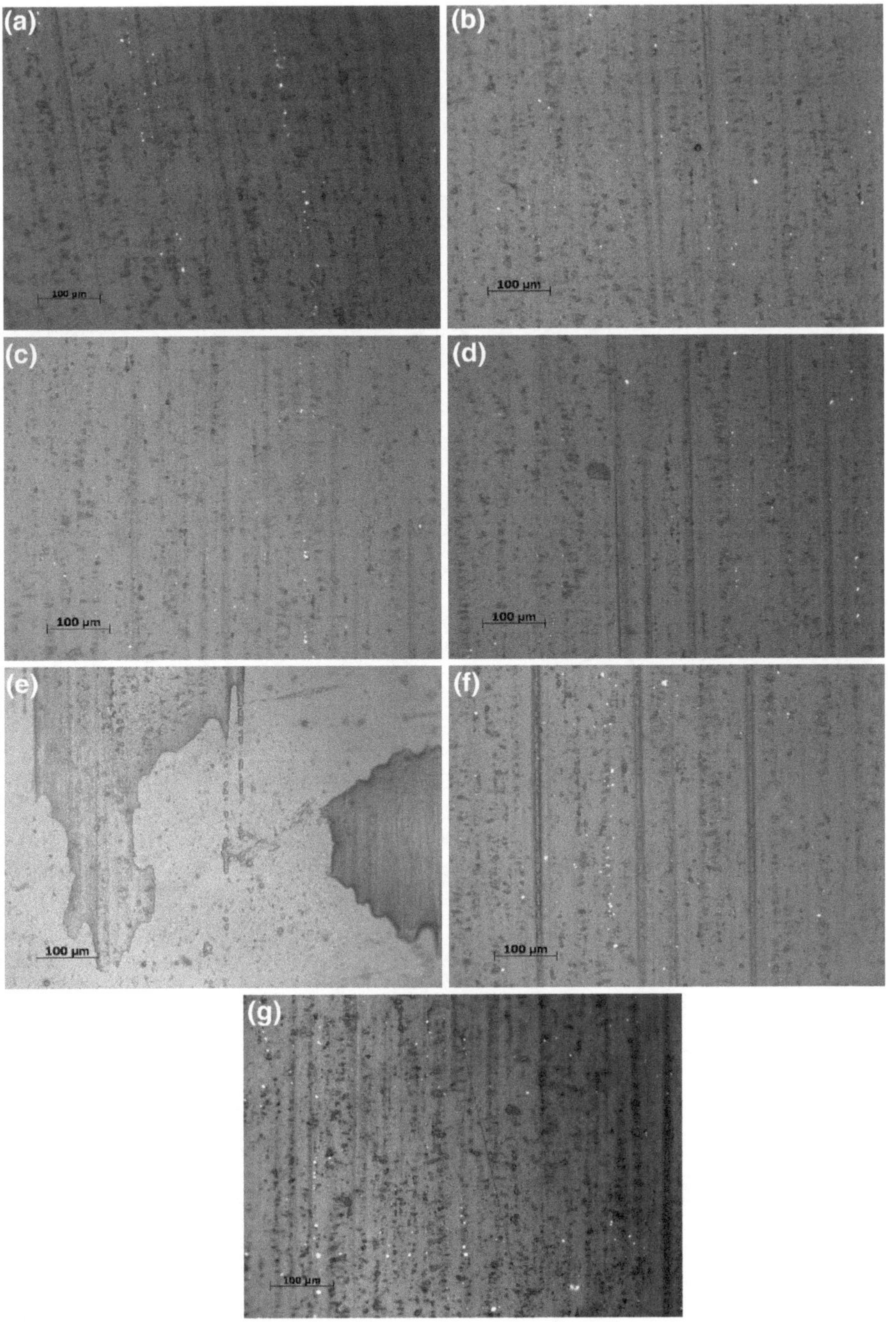

Fig. 7.3 OM micrographs of PLA samples surface at 200 × magnification **a** PLA_C—control, **b** PLA_H—hygienized, **c** PLA_{SEtO}—sterilized with ethylene oxide, **d** $PLAS_{H2O2}$—sterilized with hydrogen peroxide plasma, **e** PLA_{SSS}—sterilized with saturated steam, **f** PLA_{SEB}—sterilized with electron beam radiation, and **g** PLA_{SGR}—sterilized with gamma radiation [23]

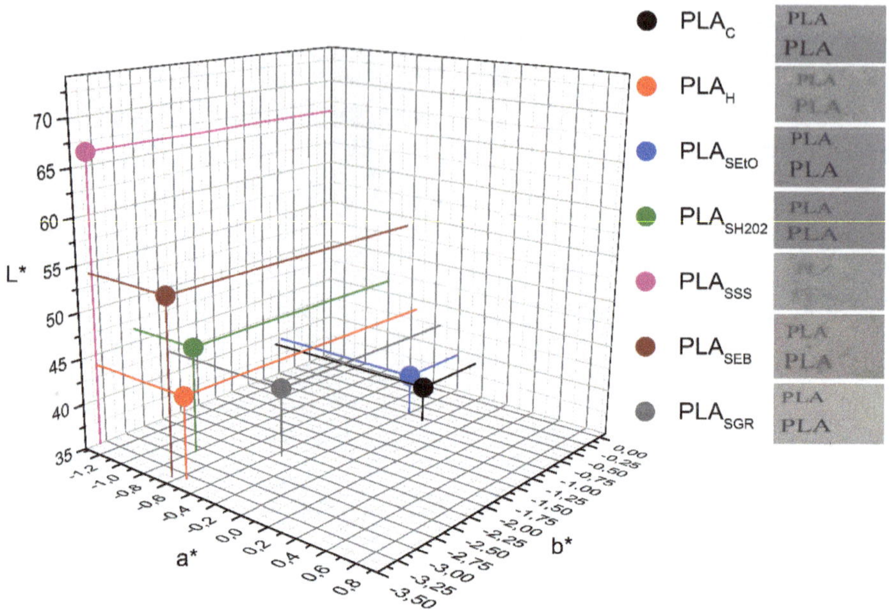

Fig. 7.4 Colorimetry by spectrophotometry of PLA samples before and after hygienization and sterilization processes. (PLA_C) control, (PLA_H) hygienized, (PLA_{SEtO}) sterilized with ethylene oxide, (PLA_{SH2O2}) sterilized with hydrogen peroxide plasma, (PLA_{SSS}) sterilized with saturated steam, (PLA_{SEB}) sterilized with electron beam radiation, (PLA_{SGR}) sterilized with gamma radiation [23]

In further studies, where different methods for polymer sterilization were applied, the use of autoclaves in most cases is not recommended for this category of materials due to the numerous morphological, physical, chemical, and thermal damage which it can cause.

References

1. Lerouge, S. Simmons.: Sterilization of biomaterials and medical devices. Woodhead Publishing Limited, Cambridge (2012)
2. Hofmann, S., Stok, K.S., Kohler, T., Meinel, A.J., Muller, R.: Effect of sterilization on structural and material properties of 3-D silk fibroin scaffolds. Acta Biomater. **10**, 308–317 (2014)
3. Zajko, S., Klimant, I.: The effects of differents sterilization procedures on the noptical polymer oxygen sensors. Sens. Actuators B Chem. **177**, 86–93 (2013)
4. Kulaga, E., Ploux, L., Roucoules, V.: Effect of ageing and sterilization on plasma multilayer system. Polym. Degrad. Stab. **116**, 1–13 (2015)
5. Ratner, B.D., Hoffman, A.S., Schoen, F.J., Lemons, J.E.: Biomaterials science: an introduction to materials in medicine, 3rd edn. Academic Press, Amsterdam (2013)

6. Miller, C.H.: Cleaning, sterilization and disinfection: basics of microbial killing for infection control. J. Am. Dent. Assoc. **124**(1), 48–56 (1993)
7. Marreco, P.R., Moreira, P.da.Luz., Genari, S.C., Moraes, A.M.: Effects of different sterilization methods on the morphology, mechanical properties, and cytotoxicity of chitosan membranes used as wound dressings. J. Biomed. Mater. Res. B Appl. Biomater. **15**, 268–277 (2004)
8. Moraes, M.A. de., Weska, R.F., Beppu, M.M.: Effects of sterilization methods on the physical, chemical, and biological properties of silk fibroin membranes. J. Biomed. Mater. Res. B Appl. Biomater. **102**, 869–876 (2013)
9. Lambert, B., Martin, J.: Sterilization of Implants and Devices. In: Ratner B.D., Hoffman, A.S., Schoen, F.J., Lemons, J.E. Biomaterials science: an introduction to materials in medicine, 3rd ed. Academic Press, Amsterdam, p. 1339–1353 (2013)
10. Rediguieri, C.F., Sassonia, R.C., Dua, K., Kikuchi, I.S., Pinto, T. de. J.A.: Impact of sterilization methods on electrospun scaffolds for tissue engineering. Eur. Polym. J. **82**, 181–196 (2016)
11. Food And Drug Administration. Ethylene oxide, ethylene chlorohydrin, and ethylene glycol. Department of health, education, and welfare. Proposed maximum residue limits and maximum levels of exposure. Rockville (1978)
12. Savaris, M., Carvalho, G.de.A., Falavigna, A., Santos, V.dos., Brandalise, R.N.: Chemical and Thermal Evaluation of Commercial and Medical Grade PEEK Sterilization by Ethylene Oxide. Mat. Res. **19**(4), 807–811 (2016)
13. Massey, L.K.: The effect of sterilization methods on plastics and elastomers, 2nd edn. William Andrew Publishing, Norwich (2005)
14. Peniston, S.J., Choi, S.J.: Effect of sterilization on the physicochemical properties of molded poly(L-lactic acid). J. Biomed. Mater. Res. B Appl. Biomater. **80B**(1), 67–77 (2007)
15. Park, J.H., Navarrete, R.O., Baier, R.E., Meyer, A.E., Tannenbaum, R., Boyan, B.D., Schwartz, Z.: Effect of cleaning and sterilization on titanium implant surface properties and cellular response. Acta Biomater. **8**(5), 1966–1975 (2012)
16. Vetten, M.A., Yah, C.S., Singh, T., Gulumian, M.: Challenges facing sterilization and depyrogenation of nanoparticles: Effects on structural stability and biomedical applications. Nanomed. Nanotech. Biol. Med. **10**, 1391–1399 (2014)
17. Ahamed, M., Punshon, G., Darbyshire, A., Seifalian, A.M.: Effects of sterilization treatments on bulk and surface properties of nanocomposite biomaterials. J. Biomed. Mater. Res. B Appl. Biomater. **101**, 1182–1190 (2013)
18. American National Standard Institute. ANSI/AAMI/ISO 11137-2—Sterilization of health care products—Radiation—Part 2: Establishing the sterilization dose, United States of America (2013)
19. Dorati, R., Colonna, C., Tomasi, C., Genta, I., modena, T., Faucitano. A., Buttafava, A., Conti, B.: γ-Irradiation of PEGd, IPLA and PEG-PLGA multiblock copolymers: II. Effect of oxygen and EPR investigation. AAPS PharmSciTech. **9**(2), 718–725 (2008)
20. Murray, K.A., Kennedy, J.E., Mcevoy, B., Vrain, O., Ryan, D., Cowman, R., Higginbotham, C.L.: Effects of gamma ray and electron beam irradiation on the mechanical, thermal, structural and physicochemical properties of poly (ether-block-amide) thermoplastic elastomers. J. Mech. Behav. Biomed. Mater. **17**, 252–268 (2013)
21. Junkar, I., Kulkarni, M., Drasler, B., Rugelj, N., Mazare, A., Flasker, A., Drobne, D., Humpolicek, P., Resnik, M., Schmuki, P., Mozetic, M., Iglic, A.: Influence of various sterilization procedures on TiO_2 nanotubes used for biomedical devices. Biolectrochemistry **109**, 79–86 (2016)
22. Nam, K.W., Yoo, J.J., Koo, K.H., Yoon, K.S., Kim, H.J.: Optimal sterilization method for the zirconia/alumina composites used for total hip replacements. J. Biomed. Mater. Res. B Appl. Biomater. **90**, 962–966 (2009)
23. Savaris, M., Santos, V. dos., Brandalise, R.N.: Influence of different sterilization process on the properties of commercial poly(lactic acid). Mat. Sci. Eng. C. **69**, 661–667 (2016)

Chapter 8
Biomaterials: Degradation and Effects on Living Tissue

Besides the already explained biocompatibility concept of Chap. 2, the cytotoxicity of the biomaterial should be an additional concept to be explored so as to elucidate the body of knowledge involving interface interactions between tissues/biomaterial for the in vivo condition.

The evaluation of biocompatibility is a complex process that involves performing in vitro and in vivo tests directed to the evaluation of cytotoxicity, allergenic responses, irritation, inflammation, and systemic and chronic toxicity [1]. Cytotoxicity is usually performed by making use of immortalized cell lines, able to be analyzed in qualitative form on the basis of morphological examination of cells damage and growth when in direct or indirect contact with materials [2].

In accordance with the ISO 10993 Standard-5 "Biological Evaluation of Medical Devices" (2009) [3], in vitro toxicity may be performed through three categories of tests: extract test, direct contact test, and indirect contact test. The choice of the category depends on the nature, location, and purpose of the utilization of the material. Based on the choice made are selected samples' preparation methods, culture cells as well as the way in which cells are exposed to the material or to the extract.

In the same way that a few concepts should be very clear, their understanding should make it possible that interdisciplinary teams constituted by medical doctors, engineers, biologists, veterinarians, pathologists, and pharmacists among other professionals once they are aware of the knowledge, could select, implant, and evaluate the biomaterial behavior in the receptor in which it is to be used.

Most of materials possess some kind of interaction with the environment that could compromise its use due to the deterioration of its properties, a phenomenon known as degradation [4].

The performance of the biomaterial to be implanted can be analyzed under various aspects: physical chemical, physiological besides its interactions with the body as a whole (tissues, organ,s and systems) [5].

When implanted, biomaterials contact body fluids that due to their chemical constitution can cause/generate a harsh environment to the biomaterial (Table 8.1).

V. dos Santos et al., *Engineering of Biomaterials*, Topics in Mining, Metallurgy and Materials Engineering, DOI 10.1007/978-3-319-58607-6_8

Table 8.1 Ionic concentrations of human tissue fluid and blood plasma [6]

Ion	Human tissue fluid* (mM)	Human blood plasma* (mM)
Na^+	142.0	142.0
HCO_3^-	4.2	27.0
K^+	5.0	5.0
HPO_4^{2-}	1.0	1.0
Mg^{2+}	1.5	1.5
Cl^-	147.8	103.0
Ca^{2+}	2.5	2.5
SO_4^{2-}	0.5	0.5

*pH between 7.2–7.4 at 37 °C, $P = 1$ atm

When in contact with such fluids the biomaterial should be biocompatible, do not produce an adverse biological response, do not lead to systemic effect and be nontoxic, carcinogenic, antigenic, or mutagenic [4].

When the biomaterial shows reactivity and undergoes degradation in contact with living tissue, the byproducts generated in the degradation can accumulate in tissues and trigger unfavorable reactions [7].

8.1 Biomaterial-Receptor and Receptor-Biomaterial Interactions

The distinct applications of different kinds of materials can trigger different responses in the receptor. These different responses, based on the interaction of the kinds of materials with tissues, circulating blood, and requirements of application are the subject matter of the present chapter considering the various classifications of materials. A further aspect which should be considered on the same subject, besides the biomaterial, interface, application, requirement, is the receptor characteristics, such as age, sex, health status among others, as evidenced in an in vivo test [5].

The response of tissues and cells toward the presence/action of the biomaterial can be determined through surface phenomena resulting from the biomaterial-tissues interface and under the aspect of residence time. This phenomenon occurs through a sequence of events involving adhesion, migration and cellular differentiation [5].

The biological processes involved in the tissue response are influenced by factors related to the implant such as [8, 9]:

- Dead space created between tissue/implant.
- Trauma resulting from the implantation and consequent inflammation.
- Soluble agents released by the implant/ions.
- Insoluble material particle released by the implant resulting from wear.

- Chemical interactions of biological molecules with the implant surface.
- Changes in the distribution of forces in tissues caused by the difference in modulus of elasticity between implant and neighboring tissue.
- Implant movement in the implanted location resulting from the lack of interaction between living tissue and the biomaterial.

A surgical implant process may be followed by the triggering of different responses in the receptor resulting from foreign matter, which can lead to inflammation and consequently trigger the cure of aggression in the case of biocompatible biomaterials. It is following an inflammation that living tissues react when in contact with a foreign body, this body being able to cause aggressions resulting from its presence as well as from degradation products originating from the material itself or from the sterilization process [7].

The inflammatory response resulting from implantation and tissue injury comprises an acute initial phase and a chronic phase. The acute phase lasts from hours to days and is responsible for fluids and protein exudation and by a neutrophilic reaction. In the acute phase, there is provisional formation of the matrix and cleaning of the injury location, vessel swelling, with excess blood flowing to the injury location. Chronic inflammation is less uniform than the acute one and the response to the injury cicatrization is dependent on injury size and degree. This phase is characterized by the presence of monocytes, macrophages, and lymphocytes, besides the proliferation of blood vessels and conjunctive tissue to restructure the affected region [10].

After the implantation a tissue/biomaterial interface is created and unspecific adsorption of blood and blood tissue fluid at the implant surface is induced. The degree and extension of the response of the foreign body depend on the material properties, such as: composition, time of contact, degradation rate, morphology, porosity, roughness, shape, size, sterility, and surface chemistry [7].

Biomaterials which are inert and have suitable interaction characteristics with the tissue lead to minimum inflammation, creating just a capsule of fibrous conjunctive tissue of variable thickness, the thickness being related to the mechanical trauma caused to the interface. It could be observed that the smaller the trauma, the smaller the layer thickness [7].

There are four local signs of rejection or inflammation shown by the tissue: heat leading to increased temperatures, blushing expressed by reddening, tumor shown by swelling, and pain [7].

Even biocompatible materials can trigger fibrous tissue formation. Fibrous tissue can assume several thicknesses which are dependent on the kind and properties of the material, the function to which it has been designed, hygienization, and sterilization processes, release of by-products and/or microparticles by the implant, besides its movement.

In a case study by Campos et al. [11] on the histological evaluation of the use of poly (methyl methacrylate) (PMMA) in Wistar rats, the foreign body evaluation generated by the application was performed using the classification by Duranti et al. [12] (Table 8.2).

Table 8.2 Duranti classification for foreign body reaction evaluation

Grade	Duranti classification
I	Slight reaction with a few inflammatory cells
II	Clear inflammatory reaction with one or two giant cells
III	Fibrous tissue with inflammatory cells, lymphocytes, and giant cells
IV	Granuloma with encapsulated implants and clear foreign body reaction

Adapted [11, 12]

Aiming at reducing the adverse effects of the receptor resulting from the use of biomaterials, the biocompatible materials the function of which is to replace the damaged tissue by promoting mechanical support under the lowest possible biological response have recently provided the actual regeneration of functional tissue with focus on the biological aspect [4]. In the search for implant increased useful life and improvement in tissues-biomaterial interaction, the attention is drawn to the development of biodegradable materials, and more recently, to the utilization of materials which actively participate in the recovery process, operating in the tissue in a specific way by stimulation at the cellular level (biomimetic materials) [13].

8.2 Behavior of the Material in the in Vivo Condition, Applications, and Requirements—Case Studies

8.2.1 Metallic Materials

The main metals and their alloys, when employed as biomaterials, develop an adherent and oxide-protecting layer on their surface. These materials when submitted to mechanical efforts can break this layer, thus exposing the metallic surface. The biological environment, where they are inserted is chemically very harsh and could lead to degradation (corrosion).

Corrosion products are responsible for biocompatibility compromising which should be localized and systemic. The pH value and the presence of proteins jeopardize metallic implants corrosion so that this phenomenon can be inhibited or accelerated [14].

Corrosion may be accelerated by ions in solution, present in body fluids (Table 8.1). Such ions influence bacterial adhesion mechanisms by toxicity or allergy to the released metallic ions. These fluids have a pH between 7.3 and 7.4; however, the pH body fluid may fall to 3–4 when there is inflammation caused by surgery or injury, due to inflammatory cells secretions. Combined with high blood pressure rise resulting from inflammation or caused by ions deposit, the human body constitutes a harsh environment for any implant, with possibility of cellular material and debris which adhere on implants. Debris are particles generated by the wear of implant components which stimulate osteolysis (Fig. 8.1), a biological

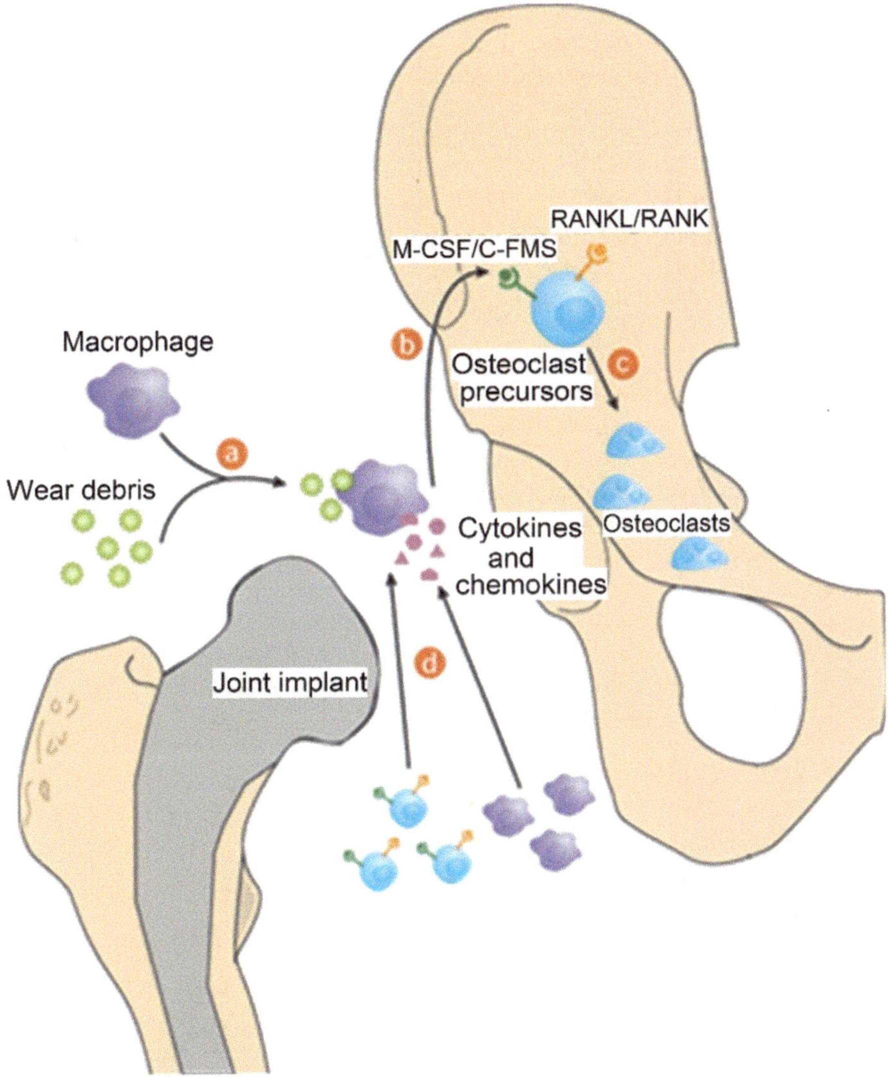

Fig. 8.1 Processes that lead to debris particle-induced osteolysis. **a** The cells take up debris via phagocytosis and secrete cytokines and chemokines in response. **b** One of these secreted cytokines, macrophage colony-stimulating factor 1 (CSF1, M-CSF), activates colony-stimulating factor 1 receptor (CSF1 R, C-FMS, CD115) on osteoclast precursors. **c** When M-CSF is present with another factor, receptor activator of NF-KB ligand (RANKL, TNFSF11), osteoclast precursors differentiate into bone-resorbing osteoclasts. **d** RANKL activates tumor necrosis factor receptor superfamily member 11a (TNFRSF11 A, RANK, CD265) and is produced by other cells such as T lymphocytes. In addition to promoting osteoclast generation, the cytokines, and chemokines secreted by the macrophage also attract additional macrophages, osteoclast precursors, and other proinflammatory cells to the area [16]

process where cells from the own body immune system attack and phagocyte the prosthesis-supporting bone. This immune system local response consumes the bone and loosens the components, causing relevant functional breakdowns in arthroplasties [6, 15].

The more corrosion-resistant stainless steels normally cause chronic allergy and toxic reactions in the receptor body, these being diagnosed only after a long postsurgery period [17–19].

Corrosion resistance should be such that metallic ions release from a metallic implant is reduced under adverse conditions of the body and is kept at a sufficiently low level for a service time period (more than 30 years) under normal physiological conditions [15].

Among the most widely corrosion forms found in metallic implants are highlighted corrosion by pitting and crevice and by wear (Fig. 8.2). Corrosion by pitting is extremely localized and is characterized by the formation of deep, small diameter cavities in the metals exposed to media-containing aggressive ions such as chloride. Crevice corrosion occurs in gaps between the metallic material in contact with another component, metallic or not. It could start, for example, at the space created by screw fixation of a metal plate. In these environments, chemical species diffusion is hindered, however, once they enter, they stay stationary, promoting changes in this space. If this process is started, the oxygen present in the gap is consumed, acidifying the solution and giving rise to corrosion. On the other hand, corrosion by wear is the result of damages produced by metallic components under direct

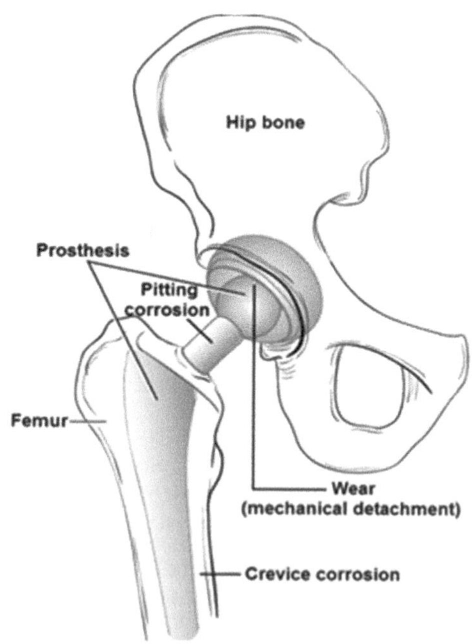

Fig. 8.2 Kinds of corrosion occurring in total prosthesis of the hip

physical contact, in the presence of vibratory movements and repeated loads, damaging the material surface, and fostering fractures build up [14, 20].

Brooks et al. [21] submitted 316L stainless steel samples to simulated inflammatory conditions. The assessment of the samples after the immersion period evidenced localized corrosion in areas susceptible to crevices at the 316L surface. This study demonstrated that care should be taken when using 316L in multi-component devices where deep crevices are susceptible to be found at component joints.

8.2.2 Ceramic Materials

On the whole, ceramic materials have fair resistance to degradation due to their high chemical stability and superior biocompatibility to metals for several applications and excellent tribological properties [14].

Among the extremes of stability and intended degradation are a small group of ceramic biomaterials, the glasses and glass ceramic materials having in their composition Ca, Si, Na, P, and O. These materials exhibit selective surface dissolution involving the release of Ca and P, but the reaction ceases due to the stable SiO_2 surface layer. This is an interesting phenomenon resulting from the ability of these surfaces to link to the bone since they have similar compositions [14].

The alumina used in prostheses of the hip should be polished in order to allow high degree of sphericity and low attrition coefficient. The presence of alumina grains larger than 4 μm and having irregular sizes distribution affect the attrition coefficient favoring abrasion and grains pullout. The attrition coefficient of alumina–alumina surfaces tends to lower with time due to the rise in alumina surface energy, a fact that benefits biological molecules adsorption. These molecules work as a liquid coating for the surfaces, reducing contact between them [22].

In a case study, a 63-year-old woman was submitted to total hip arthroplasty for the treatment of corticosteroid-induced osteonecrosis. For the arthroplasty non-cemented implants were used containing hip heads and alumina acetabulum. Eight years after surgery, the patient's implants had osteolytic lesions about the acetabular cup and greater trochanter, as can be observed by X-rays (Fig. 8.3). Abundant ceramic wear particles and a diffuse macrophagic and lymphoplasmacytic infiltrate were revealed on histologic analysis of the osteolytic tissues after staining with hematoxylin and eosin. The authors postulate that this wear and microscopic damage of the alumina liner generated sufficient phagocytosable alumina particles to elicit a macrophage response. They found abundant alumina wear particles within the macrophages that were involved in inflammation and osteolysis. In addition, most of the alumina particles were <5 μm in diameter, which is a particle size suitable for phagocytosis by macrophages.

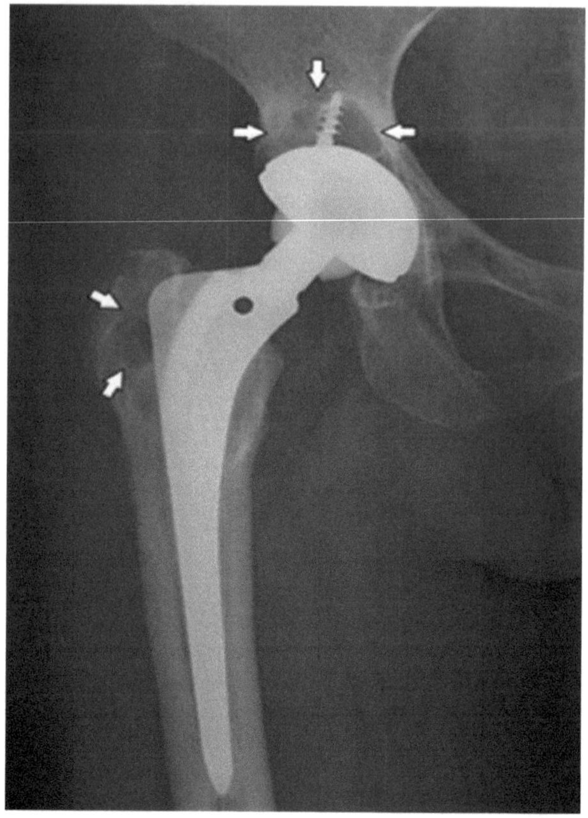

Fig. 8.3 Anteroposterior radiograph of the *right* hip, showing expansive, geographic osteolytic lesions about the acetabular cup and greater trochanter (*arrows*) eight years after alumina-on-alumina total hip arthroplasty [23]

8.2.3 Polymeric Materials

Polymeric materials used as biomaterials can, by degrading resulting from environmental action, exposure time, and application requirements, exhibit altered properties, with the consequent change in performance.

There are factors determining the inflammatory response and the degradation rate of a polymeric material when contacted with living tissue, factors deserving being highlighted comprising: implant location, chemical composition, crystallinity, and morphology of the biomaterial. The implant location should be of low vascularization (vital activity) and of low-mechanical requirement since high vascularization and strong mechanical requirement speed the degradation process. One of the factors related to chemical composition can be chirality, which enables the synthesis of enantiomer compounds giving rise to a family of polymers and copolymers of different proportions where crystallinity can be altered. Still referring to crystallinity the space distribution of polymer chains influences in water absorption rate, consequently in the onset of the hydrolysis process. As for morphology, porosity, and geometry are determinant factors as regard degradation rate [24].

Polymeric biomaterials' degradation may occur in a desirable or an undesirable way. The undesirable way refers to polymeric materials that perform a function for prolonged periods, for this class of materials degradation should not occur in a short period since the need to remain in the living tissue is for longer periods. On the other hand, when a polymeric material designed for drug release is desired, degradation is a need and it is expected to occur after days or months [25, 26].

A polymer functional period, that is, the period during which it is able to perform its functions is the most important measurement of its properties when it comes to biomaterials. For biodegradable polymers the "disappearance period" characterized by the period after which the material is completely degraded and loses mass is also important. At this moment loss of functionality is evidenced and degradation products appear which can lead to biocompatibility issues. In order to assure the right application for a polymer its functional period, disappearance period, and degradation products release rate should be characterized and monitored [25].

In the design of a biomaterial it is important to consider the kind of reaction that a certain polymer material could perform and as a result have its properties altered. It should be emphasized at this stage of the study, that high-density polyethylene by degrading in certain environments cross links and/or cyclizes and consequently its properties, for a certain exposure time, are augmented (tensile strength, modulus of elasticity, thermal stability, and chemical resistance). Depending on exposure time and environmental requirements, other degradation mechanisms can be triggered leading to loss of properties. For polypropylene, due to the presence of a tertiary carbon for every two carbons, the degradation process is by chain scission (scission-ß) and at a lower proportion by cross linking. Main chain scission leads to mechanical and thermal property losses with higher exposure times. Polymers such as polycarbonate (PC), poly(ethylene terephthalate) (PET), and poly (lactic acid) (PLA) degrade by hydrolysis, with release of by-products which can or cannot be assimilated by the natural receptor's cycles.

According to Proikakis et al. [27], the hydrolysis process is dictated by four basic parameters: rate constant, amount of absorbed water, diffusion coefficient of the chain fragments within the polymer and degradation products solubility. This process can also be influenced by parameters such as structure, molar mass, and its distribution and crystallinity as is the case for PLA, for example, besides the shape of its samples, thermal, and mechanical history (including processing) [28].

Hydrolytic degradation of a solid polymer matrix can occur through either of two alternative processes: (1) surface/core or heterogeneous erosion or (2) mass (matrix center) or homogeneous erosion. When the ongoing process is heterogeneous, polymer degradation occurs at different rates at the surface and in the interior due to the difference in water absorption in these regions, being quicker at the surface than in the interior or quicker in the interior than at the surface. In the homogeneous process, the matrix is slowly degraded and water absorption by the system is much quicker than polymer degradation. Thus, all of the system is quickly hydrated and the polymer chains are cleaved throughout the material [27].

The degradation process is dynamic, since degradation can be influenced by the characteristics of the material and further, degradation can lead to changes in its properties. For example, PLLA crystallinity increases during degradation since the degradation rate is higher in the amorphous than in the crystalline regions of the polymer leading to reduced degradation rate throughout time. On the other hand, the generation of acid monomers (lactic acid) can reduce local pH and result in increased degradation, known as autocatalysis [4]. It should be pointed out that due to lactic acid isomerism, the lactide can be found under three combinations, viz., L-lactide, D-lactide, and meso-lactide [29].

Jong et al. [30] report that amorphous (PLA) (PDLLA) hydrolytic degradation tends to occur homogeneously, being quicker in the matrix interior than at the surface. This results from the fact that the exit of degradation products (oligomers) from the matrix interior is hindered and ultimately contributes to autocatalysis and consequent degradation acceleration in its interior.

Bioresorption by the living beings body occurs when degradation products and by-products are endowed with characteristics of organic metabolites, especially acids of the Krebs Cycle. For PLA in vivo resorption and metabolization occur due to the obtention of lactic acid as a degradation product and in the body lactic acid is converted into pyruvic acid that in the presence of acetyl coenzyme A releases carbon dioxide (CO_2) and decomposes into citrate. On its turn citrate is inserted into the citric acid cycle also known as Krebs Cycle and ultimately results in CO_2 and water (H_2O), these being removed by urine and breathing [24].

By considering the different aspects which should be evaluated regarding interface interactions between tissues/biomaterial in the in vivo condition, one further kind of degradation known as "*Environmental Stress-cracking*"(ESC) should be pointed out. ESC is defined as "a phenomenon in which a polymer is degraded by a chemical agent while being under the effect of mechanical stress." However other authors define it as "the simultaneous action of stress and contact with a specific fluid." The first definition specifies the action of the chemical agent, while the second one relates only to the contact with the fluid, which can cause a plasticizing localized effect. ESC is a degradation process which combines two effects: mechanical stress and contact with a fluid. It is credited that 15% or more of all failure problems in polymeric parts result from stress-cracking. In stress-cracking the fluid is not the agent at the origin of the chemical attack to the polymer the fluid is preferably adsorbed at the polymer sites under high extensional stress (sites having residual stress resulting from processing, cracks or the end of a fracture). After being adsorbed, the fluid reduces interactions among polymer chains resulting in a localized effect of chains plasticization or disentanglement, thus promoting in the plasticized region a concentration of stress relaxation, leading to the propagation of possible cracks. With the increase in crack, adsorption of more fluid is possible to occur in this region and the effect will be slow and gradually intensified until a fracture or failure occurs.

Figure 8.4 represents the propagation of cracks in materials by ESC.

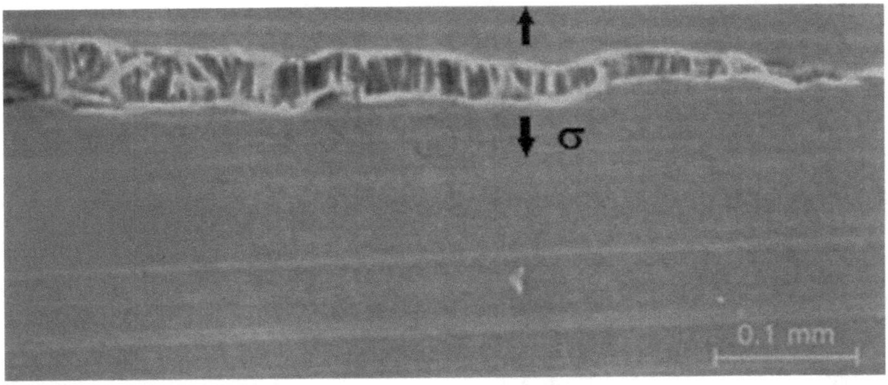

Fig. 8.4 Illustration of propagation cracks in materials by ESC. Adapted [31]

References

1. Katti, D.S., Lakashmi, S., Langer, R., Laurencin, C.T.: Toxicity, biodegradation and elimination of polyanhydrides. Adv. Drug Deliv. Rev. **54**, 933–961 (2002)
2. Marques, A.P., Reis, R.L., Hunt, J.A.: The biocompatibility of novel starch-based polymers and composites: in vitro studies. Biomaterials **23**(6), 1471–1478 (2002)
3. International Organization For Standardization. **ISO 10993-5**—Biological Evaluation of Medical Devices—Part 5: Tests for in Vitro Cytotoxicity. Geneva (2009)
4. Ratner, B.D.: Introduction: the body fights back—degradation of materials in the biological environment. In: Ratner, B.D., Hoffman, A.S., Schoen, F.J., Lemons, J.E. (eds.) Biomaterials Science—An Introduction to Materials in Medicine, 3rd edn. Academic Press, Amsterdam (2013)
5. Góes, A.M.de., Lopes, M.T.P., Maia, R.M.de.M.T., Salas, C.E.M.: Testes in Vitro com Biomateriais e Citotecnia. In: Orefice, R.L, Pereira, M.M, Mansur, H.S. (eds.) Biomateriais, Fundamentos e Aplicações. Cultura Medica, Rio de Janeiro (2006)
6. Kokubo, T., Hata, K., Nakamura, T., Yamamura, Y.: Apatite formation on ceramics, metals, and polymers induced by a CaO–SiO_2-based glass in simulated body fluid. In: Bonfield, W., Hastings, G.W., Tanner, K.E. (eds.) Bioceramics: Proceedings of the 4th International Symposium on Ceramics in Medicine. Butterworth-Heinemainn, London (1991)
7. Orefice, R.L., Pereira, M.M., Mansur, H.S.: Biomateriais, Fundamentos e Aplicações. Cultura Medica, Rio de Janeiro (2006)
8. Resende, C.M.F.de.: Testes in vivo de biomateriais e histotecnia. In: Orefice, R.L, Pereira, M.M, Mansur, H.S. (eds.) Biomateriais, Fundamentos e Aplicações. Cultura Medica, Rio de Janeiro (2006)
9. Williams, D., Cahn, R.W., Bever, M.B.: Concise Encyclopedia of Medical & Dental Materials. Pergamon Press, Oxford (1990)
10. Morais, J.M., Papadimitrakopoulos, F., Burgess, D.J.: Biomaterials/tissue interactions: possible solutions to overcome foreign body response. AAPS Journal. **12**(2), 188–196 (2010)
11. Campos, D.L.P.de., Proto, R.S., Santos, D.C.dos., Ruiz, R.de.O., Brancaccio, N., Gonella, H.A.: Histopathological evaluation of polymethylmethacrylate in rats for one year. Rev. Bras. Cir. Plást. **26**(2), 189–193 (2011)
12. Duranti, F., Salti, G., Bovani, B., Calandra, M., Rosati, M.L.: Injectable hyaluronic acid gel for soft tissue augmentation. A clinical and histological study. Dermatol. Surg. **24**(12), 1317–1325 (1998)

13. Holzapfel, B.M., Reichert, J.C., Schantz, J.T., Gbureck, U., Rackwitz, L., Noth, U., Jakob, F., Rudert, M., Groll, J., Hutmacher, D.W.: How smart do biomaterials need to be? A translational science and clinical point of view. Adv. Drug Deliv. Rev. **65**(4), 581–603 (2013)
14. Williams, D.F., Williams, R.L.: Degradative effects of the biological environment on metals and ceramics. In: Ratner, B.D., Hoffman, A.S., Schoen, F.J., Lemons, J.E. Biomaterials Science—An Introduction to Materials in Medicine, 3rd edn. Academic Press, Amsterdam (2013)
15. Sumita, M., Hanawa. T.: Failure processes in biometallic materials. Bioengineering. **9**, 131–167 (2003)
16. Lou, K.J.: Adorable implants. Analysis: targets and mechanisms—Musculoskeletal disease. Sci. Bus. Exch. **5**(25) (2012). doi:10.1038/scibx.2012.647
17. Jacobs, J.J., Skipor, A.K., Patterson, L.M., Hallab, N.J., Paprosky, W.G., Black, J., Galante, J. O.: Metal release in patients who have had a primary total hip arthroplasty. A prospective, controlled, longitudinal study. J. Bone Joint Surg. Am. **80**(10), 1447–1458 (1998)
18. Jacobs, J.J., Silverton, C., Hallab, N.J., Skipor, A.K., Patterson, L., Black, J., Galante, J.O.: Metal release and excretion from cementless titanium alloy total knee replacements. Clin. Orthop. Relat. Res. **358**, 173–180 (1999)
19. Brayda-Bruno M., Fini, M., PIerini, G., Giavaresi, G., Rocca, M., Giardino, R.: Evaluation of systemic metal diffusion after spinal pedicular fixation with titanium alloy and stainless steel system: a 36-month experimental study in sheep. Int. J. Artif. Organs. **24**(1), 41–49 (2001)
20. Walczak, J., Shahgaldi, F., Heatley, F.: In vivo corrosion of 316L stainless-steel hip implants: morphology and elemental compositions of corrosion products. Biomaterials **19**, 229–237 (1998)
21. Brooks, E.K., Brooks, R.P., Ehrensberger, M.T.: Effects of simulated inflammation on the corrosion of 316L stainless steel. Mat. Sci. Eng. C. **71**, 200–205 (2017)
22. Pereira, M.de.M., Vasconcelos, W.L., Zavaglia, C.A.de.C.: Materiais cerâmicos: ciência e aplicação como biomateriais. In: Orefice, R.L, Pereira, M.M, Mansur, H.S. (eds.) Biomateriais, Fundamentos e Aplicações. Cultura Medica, Rio de Janeiro (2006)
23. Nam, K.W., Yoo, J.J., Lae Kim, Y., Kim, Y.M., Lee, M.H., Kim, H.J.: Alumina-debris-induced osteolysis in contemporary alumina-on-alumina total hip arthroplasty. A case report. J. Bone Joint Surg. Am. American volume. **89**(11), 2499–2503 (2007)
24. Barbanti, S.H., Zavaglia, C.A.C., Duek, E.A.R.: Polímeros bioreabsorvíveis na engenharia de tecidos. Polímeros. **15**(1), 13–21 (2005)
25. Lyu, S., Untereker, D.: Degradability of polymer for implantable biomedical devices. Int. J. Mol. Sci. **10**(9), 4033–4065 (2009)
26. Adamus, A., Wach, R.A., Olejnik, A.K., Dzierzawska, J., Rosiak, J.M.: Degradation of nerve guidance channels based on a poly(l-lactic acid) poly(trimethylene carbonate) biomaterial. Polym. Degrad. Stab. **97**(4), 532–540 (2012)
27. Proikakis, C.S., Mamouzelos, N.J., Tarantili, P.A., Andreopoulos, A.G.: Swelling and hydrolytic degradation of poly(D,L-lactic acid) in aqueous solutions. Polym. Degrad. Stab. **91** (3), 614–619 (2006)
28. Belgacem, M.N., Gandini, A.: Monomers, Polymers and Composites from Renewable Resources. Elsevier, Amsterdam (2008)
29. Auras, R.A., Harte, B., Selke, S., Hernandez, R.: Mechanical, physical, and barrier properties of poly(lactide) films. J. Plast. Film Sheeting **19**, 123–135 (2003)
30. Jong, S.J., Arias, E.R., Rijkers, D.T.S., Van Nostrum, C.F., Kettenes-Van Der Bosch, J.J., Hennink, W.E.: New insights into the hydrolytic degradation of poly(lactic acid): participation of the alcohol terminus. Polymer. **42**(7), 2795–2802 (2001)
31. Deblieck, R.A.C., Van Beek, D.J.M., Remerie, K., Ward, I.M.: Failure mechanisms in polyolefines: the role of crazing, shear yielding and the entanglement network. Polymer **52**, 2979–2990 (2011)

FSC
www.fsc.org
MIX
Papier | Fördert
gute Waldnutzung
FSC® C083411

Kolibri 360 GmbH
Ferdinand-Jühlke-Straße 7
99095 Erfurt, Deutschland
produktsicherheit@kolibri360.de